Prescription Medicines, Side Effects and Natural Alternatives

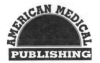

IMPORTANT NOTICE

This manual is intended as a reference volume only, not as a medical guide or a reference for self treatment. You should always seek competent medical advice from a doctor if you suspect a problem.

This book is intended as educational device to keep you informed of the latest medical knowledge. It is not intended to serve as a substitute for changing the treatment advice of your doctor. You should never make medical changes without first consulting your doctor.

Additional copies of this book may be purchased directly from the publisher. To order, please enclose $19.95 plus $3 postage and handling. Send to:

*Prescription Medicines, Side Effects
and Natural Alternatives*
American Medical Publishing
Book Distribution Center
Post Box 15196
Montclair, CA 91763

Printed in the United States of America

0 9 8 7 6 5 4 3 2 1

Table of Contents

INTRODUCTION -- A TRUE STORY

Fifty-two-year-old John Locken of Minneapolis awoke one night in bed screaming out in pain. The unbearable agony was coming from an unlikely source -- his big toe. But the pain was so bad, Locken was certain he would either pass out or die unless he got some kind of immediate help and relief. He asked his wife, Pam, to call an ambulance. Pam offered to drive him to the emergency room instead, but John's pain was so bad he knew he would have to be carried out on a stretcher. There was no way he would be able to walk far enough to get into his own car.

So Pam dialed 911 and 20 agonizing minutes later John was being rushed to the emergency room of a nearby hospital. The attending physician quickly determined the cause of John's pain -- gout. This is common, non-life threatening disease affecting 2 percent of the population. Gout can cause gradual or sudden swelling in the feet, especially in the toes. While gout seems like a minor problem to most, those who have experienced can tell you that the pain of gout can be simply unbelievable. That's because gout is caused by uric acid in the blood which crystallizes to form razor sharp splinters inside the foot. These razor crystals of uric acid cut into nerve and bone producing mind-numbing pain.

The doctor gave John an injection of a prescription narcotic for his immediate pain, which eased John's discomfort considerably, although the effect would be only temporary. To keep the pain from coming back, John would have to take some specific anti-inflammatory prescription drugs to counter the swelling in his toes and reduce the formation of the razor-sharp crystals inside his toes and feet.

By the time they returned home, John was woozy and feeling fairly pleasant from the narcotic pain killer he had received in the emergency room. He asked Pam to give him a dose of the anti-inflammatory drug the doctor prescribed for his gout. The doctor said he could take the medication on top of the pain killer without fear of a negative interaction. Pam brought John a glass of water and the pill for his gout. John dutifully swallowed it and prepared for bed.

Within minutes of settling down, however, more frightening events began to happen in John's body. He began convulsing violently, his body shaking hard enough to rock the entire bed. He fell out of bed onto the floor. John also began vomiting at the same time his body continued to shake violently. He was having a major seizure and his wife dialed 911 for the second time on that difficult night.

The ambulance arrived again and strapped John into a rolling caught, and once again he was on his way to the emergency room. Except this time, John would not arrive alive. John died before the ambulance could get him to the hospital. Upon his arrive in the emergency room, the doctor who had treated him just earlier was stunned to see him come back, DOA -- dead on arrival this time.

An autopsy was performed and it was determined that John's cause of death was the medication he had taken to relieve his gout. The medication is very common and prescribed to millions of people around the world every year. The drug is indomethacin. For most people, the drug is safe and does what it is supposed to do -- relieve the pain and swelling of gout.. But for John, the pill was a death sentence. He may have been allergic to it. But whatever the case, he died not from a minor disease of the foot, but from the very medicine that was supposed to make him feel better.

John's death went unreported in the daily newspaper the next day. The cause of death on his death certificate was listed as "seizure" but made no mention of the drug he had taken that had produced the tragic outcome in the first place. If John would have been murdered, died in a car accident, or had succumbed to flames in a burning house, his story would almost certainly have been covered by at least once local media source, if not all of them.

But John's death by prescription drug was just one more of many thousands that no one would ever hear about, except for close family and friends. The general public -- many of which might be taking the very same drug the next day -- would never hear about the way John died.

Maybe you will be prescribed the same drug John took for what he thought was a minor ailment, easily treated by a common drug manufactured by a major drug company, and prescribed to him by a trusted, licensed doctor. Maybe the next time you take a pill, you won't be alive to see the sunrise the next morning. It might be the same pill John trustingly took, or it may be one of several thousands of other medication you have in your medicine cabinet right now.

In one of those pills can kill you. In this book, you'll find out why, and how to protect yourself.

Chapter One

PRESCRIPTION DRUGS -- OUR BIGGEST KILLER?

More than 25,000 Americans are murdered every year. Twice as many, about 50,000 people, die in terrible car accidents every year. Prostate cancer takes the lives of about 40,000 men in America annually, and 52,000 people die from heart attacks. The dread disease AIDS claims tens of thousands lives per year in America, and millions worldwide.

We hear about all of the above on a daily basis. You can't pick up a newspaper or turn on the television without hearing about least one kind of tragic death from these major killers. Indeed, the media report deaths from disease, murder and accidents so frequently, we almost take it for granted. But because we also know about the dangers of driving, disease and crime, the majority of us take steps to make sure we lessen our own chances of having to confront all of the above. When we get in a car, we fasten our seat belts, obey traffic signs, and do our best to "watch out for the other guy." Most people do what they can to eat right and avoid bad habits, such as smoking, to prevent chances of heart attacks, cancer and other diseases. Smart people take precautions to avoid contracting HIV and other sexually transmitted diseases.

But if we were to tell you that there is probably something in your house right now which is four times more likely to kill you than a murderer, or twice as likely to kill you as a car accident, and 100 times as likely to kill than AIDS? Furthermore, what if we were to tell you that you have no idea that this thing in your home is dangerous -- and that you probably actually believe just the opposite is true about this major killer -- you have been told and have accepted that it is safe, and will even make you more healthy than you are now.

Well, there is very likely a major killer in your home, and it's as close as your medicine cabinet. The fact is that prescription drugs, and even many common over-the-counter drugs you can buy in any drugstore or health food store, kill at least 100,000 people per year, and most likely, many more. That's four times as many people who die by murder, and twice as many people who die in car accidents every year. In addition to 100,000 deaths, about 2 million more people suffer serious and/or permanent injury caused by a prescription drug they believed to be safe. Sometimes the people that die are the lucky ones. Many of the 2 million injured suffer permanent brain damage, loss of use all or parts of their bodies, and worse.

Some believe the estimate of 100,000 prescription drug caused deaths is actually a very conservative estimate. The numbers could be much higher -- from 200,000 to 400,000 deaths per year. Getting the exact numbers is difficult for some very troubling reasons you will read about in just a minute.

But for now, think about this: When is the last time you remembered seeing a story in the newspaper about a person who died or was sickened from taking a medicine prescribed to him or her by their own doctor? We read about murders and deadly car accidents every day -- but we rarely, and almost never, do we read about something that is killing more people much more frequently, much more tragically, and with greater efficiency. People die in car accidents every day, and your local newspaper or TV station will tell you about it every time. If someone gets murdered in your town or neighborhood, reporters will be right on the spot to let you know. But if 1,2, 5 or even ten people in your town die from a prescription drug will there be a reporter on the scene to let you know about it? Will you see a article in the newspaper about it or a spot about it on the local news? The answer is no, and almost never!

There is something terribly wrong with this picture. It seems only common sense that the bigger, more deadly killer would get and deserve more media attention so that more people could be aware of it, and thus take steps to avoid it. But while we are all constantly urged to buckle up our seat belts, there is nothing but silence on the many thousands of deaths -- more than 275 every day -- resulting from people who take prescription drugs given to them by their own doctor.

This is a fact: one person is dying every two minutes in America by taking a prescription drug prescribed to them buy their own trusted doctor!

If prescription drugs are more deadly than car accidents or murderers, why aren't we all more aware of it? Why don't we hear more about it? Why isn't there some kind of ongoing public safety campaign to address this serious problem? Why do so many people have to die needlessly by a killer that most of us are simply not even aware of?

All of the above are very good questions, and the answers are disturbing. Let's look at why there seems to be a true conspiracy of silence about the dangers of prescription drugs.

THE BIG DRUG COMPANIES

First of all, consider the fact that the American prescription drug industry -- the giant pharmaceutical companies -- is the most profitable industry in the world. Drug companies make more money than banks, more money than oil companies, more money than Ford or GM, more money than anybody. Drug companies spend billions of dollars on advertising and promotion -- some $10 billion every year. This advertising is directed at both doctors, and directly to the public. Drug companies spend billions promising better health and an enhanced lifestyle if only you'll convince your doctor to prescribe them to you, and if you take them as directed. It is said that tobacco`-- cigarettes, cigars and chewing tobacco -- is the only product on the market that can kill you if used as directed. But that is certainly not true. The fact is, more than 100,000 people die every year if they take drugs prescribed to them by doctors, and take them exactly as directed.

You see, we're not talking about deaths that result from people who abuse prescription drugs, or take them improperly, or not as directed. No, we're talking about prescription drugs that kill if taken exactly as directed! Even though drug companies are required to list the possible side effects and dangers of their products, this latter deadly possibility is skillfully placed in the fine print, and rarely spoken of by the very doctors who are getting paid to dole them out to their patients. The drug companies are in the business of developing and manufacturing drugs, but they are also in the business of making money. As we will argue throughout this book, it is the profit motive that is making what should be a life-saving and health generating industry into a make-money-at-any-cost industry, whether it kills tens of thousands of people or not.

THE DOCTORS: COVERING THEIR BACKS?

And that brings us to another possible reason why death by prescription drugs is so little known. The doctors themselves have no incentive to admit that the very drugs they prescribe can sometimes kill. Today in America, doctors live in daily fear of being sued for malpractice and doing harm to patients. Doctors pay enormous fees for malpractice insurance coverage, and those fees are getting higher every year. Every time a doctor injures or kills a patient, they face the prospect of a costly lawsuit, any one of which could end their career, or at the very least, drive them to financial ruin.

Doctors also have an image and reputation to maintain. No

doctor wants to go out of his way to advertise how many patients die under his or her own care. Doctors can hardly be blamed for this attitude. They have a certain legitimate excuse for downplaying their failures and emphasizing their successes. Doctors are human beings. Doctors are not perfect. Modern medicine and science is not perfect. That means people are going to die no matter what, even when a doctor does all the right things. If all doctors were held responsible for every patient that dies under their care, there would soon be no doctors at all, and we can all agree that's not a good thing. Doctors are also blameless in that they, too, are only following instructions as dictated by the manufacturers of drugs. The family doctor or the specialist you see in a clinic is not the inventor of the prescription drug, but merely the highly trained agent charged with doling them out properly to patients. Drugs are the weapons provided to doctors who must properly diagnose diseases, and then match up the right disease with the right drug. Sometimes the doctors get it wrong and prescribe the wrong drug. Most often the harm is none or minimal.

So it's worth repeating that doctors can not be entirely blamed for the fact that a lot of people are dying from prescription drugs.. Doctors are only doing their best to help sick people get better, to cure disease, and improve the lives and health of all the people they treat every day. But doctors, like anyone else, are not only subject to unavoidable error -- they can also succumb to lapses in ethics. Doctors are also not immune to such common human failings as greed and the desire to make as much money as possible in any way they can. Doctors also tend to protect their own. That is, organizations, such as the American Medical Association and similar professional associations actively protect and shield doctors from criticism and blame. Such organizations do a pretty good job of policing themselves, but they strongly resist any outside independent effort to criticize or take action against them. For example, the FDA has set up an adverse drug reaction reporting system which asks doctors to report all incidents of harm or death that results from the drugs they prescribe. The problem is, the system is only voluntary. Doctors actually shun the system and former Food and Drug Administration commissioner David Kesslersaid that just 1% of serious negative drug reaction events are reported through this system. This is true despite the fact that the FDA has made it easy and free of disciplinary action against doctors if they make a report. Yet doctors ignore making reports 99% of the time. Kessler said the doctors themselves are conditioned by their own professional culture not to make such reports. Doctors are very bad at admitting error, even when they can do so anonymously, and without fear of punishment.

So here we have two explanations for why most of us are unaware of the deadly potential of prescription drugs -- money-making pharmaceutical companies who don't want the public to know that their products can cause death, and doctors who have no incentive or desire in letting it be known that the drugs they prescribe sometimes kill their own patients.

YOUR OWN GOVERNMENT

A third problem is flaws in our own government. The agency charged with monitoring the safety of prescription drugs is the FDA -- the Food and Drug Administration. The immediate drawback to this is, of course, is obvious. The FDA is just that -- a large, bureaucratic government agency that moves as slow as a drunken turtle, and is weighted down with endless rules, regulations, paperwork and a budget that is too small to handle all the work it is expected to do. Every year, the FDA is responsible for examining and approving or rejecting literally thousands of drugs. At the same time, it takes the FDA an average of 16 months to make a decision on each single drug. While the FDA is trying to handle this tremendous load of work, its officials are constantly bombarded with all kinds of political pressure from politicians; it is harassed by drug company lobbyists who always want "fast track" approval for a particular drug; they are also pressured by other special interest groups, including sick people who do not want to wait 16 months for the approval of a drug they think they need right away to save their lives, or relieve them of a painful medical condition.

Again, the idea here is not to paint the FDA and its staff as being some how to "blame" or with irresponsibility when it comes to prescription drugs -- but like doctors, they get caught up in the larger games that are inevitably played around the issue of prescription drugs. The result is, to make a long story short, that the government agency which is charged with making sure our drugs are safe cannot possibly do it's job with 100% efficiency. To say that a particular drug has received "FDA approval" is simply no guarantee that the drug is safe and effective.

In a report recently issued by a government investigative agency which studied the FDA, the report's author's said:

``It's a tragedy that so many of these 100,000 deaths a year are preventable. Many of them could be avoided by more effective oversight. ... Clearly, Congress has a responsibility to give high priority to these important reforms."

The FDA itself does not deny that there is a serious problem. FDA drug chief Dr. Janet Woodcock recently said this to a congressional panel looking into problems with prescription drugs:

`We can't just sit here in Washington and receive reports (from drug makers) and know what's going on in the community. There's no doubt the toll of deaths and injuries, and the economic costs of adverse drug reactions, is really staggering." Woodcock said.

The government watchdog report also pointed out that even when drugs are tested before they are approved, the tests themselves are not rigorous and careful enough. New drugs are tested on only a few hundred to a few thousand patients before they're sold to millions, meaning rare side effects that didn't show up in small clinical trials can wind up hurting hundreds and maybe thousands of people.

A BIG PART OF THE PROBLEM -- YOU!

As you can see, there is plenty of blame to go around when considering the dangers of prescription drugs. But let's not leave out another important element of the problem: it's you me -- all of us -- the public at large. How can the ordinary man on the street be to blame for prescription drugs that can kill people? Well, the relationship is somewhat indirect, but certainly worth considering.

The fact is, the general public has come to trust blindly the powers that be in the realm of prescription drugs. People just assume that the mighty FDA is doing a perfect job all the time when it examines prescription drugs for safety. People place blind trust in their doctors. People just assume that the big drug companies -- with their armies of brilliant research scientists -- are doing not just good work, but perfect work, when they discover, research and manufacture new drugs. And for the most part, all of the above is generally true. But the problem is that no one is infallible -- not doctors, not government safety experts, and not brilliant research scientists. Furthermore, the more trust the public puts in doctors, drug manufacturers and government watchdogs, the easier it becomes for them all to become lax, get sloppy and get by with less than the highest possible standards of safety and accountability. Most people feel extremely intimidated by the vast system that supplies the world with medical drugs. They think: "What can I do? If they say this drug is safe, if my doctor prescribed it, who am I to question it. After all, not everyone can have a degree in biochemistry and medical pharmacology!"

That's true, but this does not mean that the general public must simply roll over and play helpless when it comes to their own safety, even in the arena of prescription drugs. The population in general can demand that their own government officials do a better job to police the prescription drug industry. People do not have to put blind faith in their doctors and the drugs they prescribe for them. For example, a patient can easily access all kinds of information about the drug they have been prescribed to take in a number of places. They can visit a library and research the safety level of the drug they have been prescribed to take. Just a few minutes on an Internet search engine can reveal a great deal of information about the drug in question. They can find out if other people were harmed or killed by this particular drug, and why. They can get a second opinion from another physician. They can also question their primary physician as to what his experience has been with this drug and other patients who used it.In short, you are the one who is ultimately responsible for your own safety. The more blind faith and trust you put into your government, doctor and drug company, the less accountable they are to you or anyone else who needs medicine for better health or to save a life.

NEW AGGRESSIVE DRUG ADVERTISING

Anyone who watches television cannot but help notice a new trend in the past couple of years -- suddenly our TV programs are flooded with advertisements for dozens of new prescription drugs. And they seem to promise everything. Night after night, television commercials paid for by drug companies are promising to fix or cure everything from depression and sleeplessness, to arthritis and allergy problems. You name it, they've got a drug for it, be the problem as serious as cancer, or as trivial as baldness and unattractive toenails.

The reason you never saw so many prescription drug commercials before is that, up until 1998, federal law prohibited the advertisement of prescription drugs to the general public. But after a heavy lobbying effort by big drug companies -- and a lot of big bucks campaign contributions to our senators and congressmen -- our government lifted the ban on pitching prescription drugs directly to consumers. The reason for the previous ban was based on good common sense -- prescription drugs are extremely dangerous if used without the direction of a licensed doctor. Since only doctors can prescribe prescription drugs to the general public it made no sense to advertise them to people who could not buy them over-the-count, and without a doctor's approval.

But the big drug companies had other ideas. they thought: "If we can get people to start asking their own doctors for specific drugs, we'll sell more of our products, and we'll make bigger profits."

And that's just what happened. The only problem is, the commercials which sell prescription drugs are like all advertising -- filled with hype, unrealistic promises and subtle bending of the truth. No doubt, you've seen some of the ads on TV. They feature ecstatically happy people who seem to have had their lives transformed by drug the particular ad is pushing. TV ads for prescription drugs make it seem like anything can be fixed, cured or chased away by simply swallowing a magic pill that solves all problems, with no side effects, and no threat of danger or death.

Of course, TV ads for drugs also make brief mention of potentially harmful side effects. It was just this requirement -- the disclosure of possible dangers and drawbacks of the drug -- which allowed drugs ad to appear on TV in the first place. By listing side effects, the drug industry argues, full responsibility is being taken for the potential risks involved in using a prescription drugs.

But, again, there is a problem. While TV ads for drugs do indeed list potential harmful side effects, the slickly produced ads gloss over them so fast, and with such finesse, it creates an overwhelming impression among the public that these potential dangers are all but nothing to worry about. Also, TV ads do not list all of the potential side effects, but rather, just the most common side effects. So in effect, advertisements for prescription drugs on television are literally lying by omission. They list a few common side effects, but ignore dozens, and possible hundreds of other side effects each drug is known to produce. So when you see an ad for a prescription drug on TV, you simply are not getting the full story. Instead, what you are getting is a super hyped, glamorized and only partial version of the total story and the total truth.

Even worse, many television ads for prescription drugs actually encourage dangerous behavior for people with medical conditions. For example, ads for the popular prescription allergy medications, Allegra and Claratin, often depict people hugging shaggy dogs or frolicking in fields of wild flowers, weeds and plants. For people with serious allergies, most doctors would agree that it is best to avoid those agents which trigger allergic reactions. Yet, the drug commercials show just the opposite. The message is: "If you take this drug, you are cured, and no longer have to worry about all of those things which made you sick before." The message is: "As long as you take Allegra or Claratin. you are immune to all those old problems."

But this is not true. Certainly, allergy medications such as Allegra and Claratin can be very effective in controlling allergic reactions to things like animal hair, wild flowers, pollen and dust. This does not mean, however, that 100% control can be expected, or is guaranteed. It would be a much better idea for people with allergy problems to avoid those triggers which cause allergic reactions. Drugs for allergies should be used for those occasions when adverse contacts cannot be easily avoided, or when contact is made accidentally or unawares. The message of the ads appears to be just the opposite. "Take this pill and go do whatever you want!"

Hundreds of people die every year from adverse allergic reactions. Some people cough or choke to death from contact with pollen or dust. Some people may go into allergic shock. Many of those people may be under the impression that their magical, oversold allergy medication is protecting them completely. But no drug, no matter how good, is 100% effective. In some cases, the result can be death. Admittedly, such a scenario is unlikely -- but we give this example to make a larger point. Even though drugs like Allegra and Claratin are marvelous inventions and have undoubtedly helped millions of people breath easier and live better lives, the potential for disaster remains. And the way television commercials present their products -- in this case prescription drugs -- leads to the false impression among consumers that these are actually magic pills that provide complete immunity from any and all health related problems.

Again, the drug companies would argue that many safety precautions are in place, the primary one of which is that the drug is still only used under the direction of a doctor. The side effects of the drugs are stated up front, and a doctor should be advising the patient on correct usage and of potential pitfalls of the drug. But as we have already said, doctors have little incentive to report their failures. If a patient under a doctor's care dies or is seriously harmed by a drug, the doctor is simply not going to go out of his or her way to promote what went wrong. A doctor can also deflect blame back to the drug company. To which the drug company can simply say: "We warned the consumer of the side effects. No drug is perfect!" There is also money involved. Drug companies make it financially attractive for doctors to push their drugs on their patients.

But even if a doctor does a perfect job of warning and advising a patient on the use of a particular prescription drug, the power of advertising can easily overcome those warnings. There is a saying in advertising: "Call a man a dog once and you insult him. Call him a dog a thousand times and he may start barking!" The meaning of this statement is this: constant repetition of a message makes that message more believable, even if it seems ridiculous at first. That's why you see ads and television commercials over and over again. The more they hammer away at a message, the more they break down our psychological resistance to that message. The same effect can work for prescription drug ads. Even though a doctor has warned a patient about the danger of a drug, a constant bombardment of "happy ads" can easily create an impression in the mind of the consumer that the drug is not only completely safe, but capable of transforming one's life into a kind of blissful paradise.

CONCLUSIONS

In this chapter you have learned something the vast majority of Americans are unaware of -- the fact that prescription drugs kill 100,000, and possible tens of thousands more people every year. Someone is dying every two minutes from an adverse reaction to a prescription drug. In the time is took you to read this chapter, 5 to 10 people died after taking a prescription drug. In addition to hundreds of thousands of deaths, some 2 million more people are seriously injured or permanently impaired as the result of a prescription drug. The reason that prescription drugs are not recognized as one of the biggest killers in America is complex. Drug companies who make huge profits from the sale of drugs spend more than $10 billion a year promoting drugs, and spend next to nothing warning the public about potential risks. Drug companies also engage in misleading advertising campaigns which make outright false or unrealistic claims, but which convince that vast majority of the public that most or all prescription drugs are not only safe, but the key to better health and a better life. The doctors themselves are also a part of the problem. Doctors chronically under-report and even ignore the deaths or adverse reactions to the drugs they prescribe because it is not in their professional self interest to raise public awareness to the danger. Doctors are afraid of being sued, they maintain a culture of denial, and they also profit from there relationships with the big drug companies. The government is also part of the problem because it does not have the resources or the political will to do more about the dangers of prescription drugs. Also, powerful members of the American government, from the President on down, are all lobbied heavily by the cash rich drug companies. They donate millions of dollars to political election campaigns, and many politicians are eager to grant favors to drug companies in exchange for lax enforcement of government regulations and safety standards. Finally, the public at large has itself to blame as well. People have come to expect miracles and "magic pills" from medical researchers and doctors. Such expectations are unrealistic and do nothing to pressure the drug companies, doctors and the government to do a better job of making the pharmaceutical system safer. In the last presidential election, less than half of all eligible voters exercised their right to vote. The president was elected with less than one-fourth of all the potential votes in America. American have very little interest in what their own government is doing, while large wealthy corporations, such as drug companies, are paying careful attention to who gets elected and who does not. They work hard to make sure that only those candidates favorable to drug company policies get elected. The result is a government doing little to police a major industry that is getting wealthy by producing products -- in this case prescription drugs -- that do a lot of good, but also kill tens of thousands of people per year, and sicken millions more.

Chapter Two

PROZAC -- THE "CLEAN DRUG" WITH SOME DIRTY SECRETS

NEWS ITEM:

In 1989, Joseph Wesbecker brought an assault rifle into the printing plant where he had worked in downtown Louisville, Ky., and opened fire. He his own life. At the time, he was taking Prozac.

Six years later, a jury found that there was no reason to blame the popular antidepressant drug or its manufacturer, Eli Lilly & Co., for the carnage. It was Wesbecker's mental illness, they ruled, and not the medication, that fueled his attack.

Even though the judge later discovered that a secret settlement had been reached before the case even went to the jury, the case still had "a chilling effect" on future lawsuits, says Houston attorney Arnold "Andy" Vickery. "With the exception of me, I don't know anybody who's taking on new cases against these drug companies. It's a monumental effort."

-- Source: ABC NEWS

In the next few chapters we we are not going to talk about drugs that have a high chance of killing you or someone you love We're going to focus on some selected extremely popular, common and widely prescribed drugs that can easily ruin the lives of people who take them, of kill. No doubt, many readers will be surprised to find that they may be using one of these prescription drugs right now, or you may have friends or loved ones whom you know are using these drugs. What you learn in this chapter and those that follow may surprise and disturb you and surprise you. But our advice is to for you to take in this information calmly and with an open mind. What you read here is merely "the other side the story" -- the stories the billion dollar drug manufacturers spend so much time ignoring, while at the same time spending billion upon billions promoting only the benefits. So let's start with a drug that is certainly been the most sensational, popular and one of the most widely prescribed in the past decade -- Prozac, and its close "cousin" drugs, Paxil, Zoloft.

THE TROUBLING STORY OF PROZAC

Unless you have been living in a cave for the past 10 years, you have certainly heard about the powerful new drug often touted as "a cure" for one one man's oldest and most terrible enemies -- depression. The drug is most commonly sold under the brand name of Prozac. The generic name for the drug is fluoxetine, but the full, correct chemical name for Prozac is fluoxetine hydrochloride It was developed by the pharmaceutical giant Eli Lilly, which owns the patent for Prozac.

The story of how Prozac was developed is amazing, although we'll just touch on it only very briefly here. Scientists working on drugs that affected the brain wanted a way to test the way certain chemical compounds worked on brain cells, and specifically, on brain synapses. A synapse is a nerve ending in a brain cell. Chemicals in the brain "jump" from one synapse to another as the brain carries out it's normal functioning. This is how the brain thinks, feels emotions, carries out bodily functions -- all of human experience is carried along the synapses of human brain cells.

Scientists at Eli Lilly developed a method of experimenting with brain cells that was revolutionary. They used the brains of rats -- which have strong similarities to the brains of humans -- for their test models. What they did was develop a method of isolating individual synapses from the rest of the brain so they could test exactly what was happening when they tried different kinds of chemicals on them.

The method sounds like a Frankenstein story and will seem cruel if you are a lover of rats or animals in general, but at any rate here is what they did. They removed the brains of rats and crushed them up. Then they put the crushed brain matter into a centrifuge -- a spinning machine -- which would eventually spin out the clean nerve endings -- the synapses -- or rat brains. And here is the amazing part -- this isolated brain cell was still alive! They were able to crush the brains and separate the brain cells they wanted while keeping the cells totally alive and functioning.

Once this was accomplished, it was extremely easy to test

thousands of different compounds on living, isolated rat brain cells. Specifically, what they were trying to do was find a substance that would block the flow of a natural brain chemical known as serotonin. Serotonin is what scientists call a neurotransmitter -- a chemical that transmits information along the nerve pathways of the brain. The reasons that the researchers at Eli Lily were so interested in serotonin is that it was widely believed the people who suffered from depression had abnormal flow rates of serotonin in their brains. They believed that if they could find a chemical that could block or slow down the flow of serotonin between brain cells, they would have a substance that could possibly treat or even cure depression.

So the scientists began testing thousands of different substances that would slow the flow of serotonin in the brain, and they did so with incredible patience. The great inventor Thomas Edison is well known for his perseverance because he tested more than 1,200 different substances before he finally found the right one that could be used successfully as a filament for the first light bulb. But the scientists at Eli Lilly had more luck with their goal -- on their 250th try, they found a substance that did exactly what they wanted it to do. The substance was fluoxetine oxolate, but later they discovered that a very similar substance was easier to work with -- fluoxetine hydrochloride -- and that is what Prozac is.

Interestingly, Prozac is not the first known substance or drug that was invented with the purpose of blocking serotonin uptake in brain cells. Older antidepression drugs already could do that, including a popular drug known generically as norepinephrine, but Prozac was much better because it was 200 times more effective blocking serotonin than even the best of older antidepression drugs. Also, Prozac was called a "clean drug" because it blocked serotonin with far fewer side effects.

This term --"clean drug" -- is important to our story because it is a term that caught hold with the media. The term may have been coined by a doctor and psychiatrist by the name of Peter D. Kramer, who wrote a best selling book about Prozac called Listening to Prozac. In this book, Kramer frequently praises Prozac, it's safety, and the fact that it is a "clean drug." In fact, one could almost believe that Kramer was on the Eli Lilly payroll as he wrote his book, so full of gushing acclaim and unabashed promotion of the wonders and life changing qualities Prozac has had on his patients and millions of other people.

The media picked up on Kramer's "clean drug" description and ran with it. Prozac indeed seemed to be a miracle drug. Kramer and dozens of other sources praised Prozac as not only an incredibly powerful medicine for depression, but also fantastically free of side effects. Even taking a dangerous overdose of Prozac seems to be all but impossible. Kramer says in his book: "Prozac was safer in the hands of potentially suicidal patients who might attempt to overdose on the drug. Because of the likelihood of effects on the heart, Prozac overdoses are relatively benign."

Kramer goes on to say that Prozac seems capable of "curing" all kinds of mental disorders, not just depression alone. He tells of a man who lost interest in watching naughty pornographic video tapes. He tells of businessmen and women who suddenly became more successful at their jobs because Prozac made them think quicker and with more confidence. He tells of sexual problems erased and even compulsive overeaters suddenly losing interest in eating too much and growing slender, beautiful, popular and blissfully happy.

Kramer also said that Prozac often way beyond just curing depression -- it also made people feel not only happy, but "more like the person they were supposed to be." So Prozac not only lifted the blues, it seemed capable of turning ordinary people into superhuman people -- better at making money, free of crude sexual habits, such as liking to watch dirty movies, slimmer, more confident in sexual relationships, and even more spiritually happy.

Since Prozac was introduced in 1990, the media went crazy over this new "clean drug" and the general public went even crazier. Even though Prozac was one of the most expensive "designer" drugs ever -- selling at more than $2 a pill -- millions of people rushed to their doctors and begged for a prescription. Doctors everywhere obliged them, and soon Eli Lilly was making billions upon billions of dollars on its new wonder drug -- an apparently totally safe drug with few or no side effects, which could work miracles on the lives of anyone who tried it. Even people who were not really depressed sought out Prozac for what they thought it might do for them. Big time corporate executives took Prozac hoping it would give them an edge in difficult trade negotiation and in money making abilities. People who were unlucky at love hoped Prozac would make them sexy, popular and attractive to the opposite sex everywhere. People who felt spiritually empty hoped Prozac would literally help them find God, or at least a greater understanding of what life was all about. Remember, Kramer's book and media articles from thousands of sources profiled people who claimed that Prozac had given them all of the above.

So what about Prozac? Is it really the totally safe, "clean" miracle drug that millions of people have believed it to be for the past 10 or more years? Well, there's another side to Prozac that gets very little, if no media attention, and we'll discuss this possible darker side right now.

NOT SO CLEAN?

First of all, it's worth noting that Prozac is not the first "miracle drug" which doctors, scientists and researchers have unleashed on the public, claiming it was a veritable cure-all for a dozen different mental and physical condition. You may be surprised to learn the name of some of those past "miracle" drugs. They include tobacco, caffeine, cocaine, opium, Valium, amphetamines of all kinds, addictive barbiturates of all kinds, and even marijuana.

Many famous people actively promoted the use of such miracle drugs. Less than a 100 years ago the great Sigmund Freud, a genius and the father of modern psychology, firmly believed that cocaine was not only an excellent remedy for colds, soar throats and the flu, he also heralded its psychological benefits. Freud believed cocaine was a safe and effective drug for millions of mental patients. And at first, the public believed it. Cocaine became an extremely widely prescribed and used "medicine" throughout the world. Cocaine was even made the primary ingredient in a popular drink -- Coca Cola. The "coca" refers to cocaine, and the soft drink was originally made with the substance. But it didn't take long for the public at large to catch on that the "miracle drug" cocaine was far less a miracle than a true monster. Today, cocaine is one of the most feared substances on earth, and law enforcement officials spend millions of dollars trying to keep it out of the hands of people on the streets. What was once a cure-all miracle drug is now one of humanities biggest curses.

The same phenomenon has been documented time and time again throughout history. A wonderful new drug -- usually a psychoactive drug, as is Prozac -- bursts onto the scene, is embraced by the most intelligent people of the day, only to find out a decade or so later that the substance is not all it has cracked up to be -- and often just the opposite -- an addictive scourge that ruins lives, causes death and eats away at the fabric of society.

This lesson should be reviewed in the case of Prozac. Again, we see the same pattern: the discovery of a fabulous new substance; fantastic claims of cure-all properties; testimonials to it's incredible safety and lack of side effects -- and then the slow realization that it's not all it's cracked up to be.

Certainly, it is not fair to compare Prozac with cocaine or opium -- but yet, many disturbing similarities exist between this new miracle drug and old miracle drugs that turned out not be that at all.

In fact, some very frightening stories about Prozac jumped up within months after it was introduced to the general public in 1990. They were horror stories. Some of the first people to take Prozac were suddenly involved in bizarre cases of violence, murder, suicide and all kinds of strange psychotic behavior. One of the first warning flags was raised by three Harvard teachers who published a disturbing article in the American Journal of Psychiatry in 1990 -- the year Prozac was released for public use.

Harvard researcher Martin Teicher reported that six people who were treated for depression with Prozac developed "intense, violent suicidal tendencies." after just two to seven weeks of treatment with Prozac. It was further observed that each patient lost their suicidal and violent tendencies after they were taken off Prozac. The report was alarming, but the damage to the image of Prozac was minimized after Prozac supporters rushed in to point out flaws in the study of the six people. It was noted that the patients had long histories of mental problems, and that they were also taking a number of other medications at the same time they were taking Prozac. In some cases, Prozac was the sixth medication they were on at the time. Yet, when only the Prozac was removed, the violent thoughts and intentions disappeared. But so soon did the study and any early warning flags it might have raised.

A couple of years later, sporadic reports began to crop in the media about a number of people who went on wild murderous rampages, killing several people, or killing themselves after being prescribed Prozac. For a while, there was a lot of worry among the media and general public. Time magazine even featured a giant picture of a Prozac on it's front cover as a controversy about the dangers of Prozac seemed to be gaining momentum. But again, Prozac supports rushed in with their own studies showing that the connection between Prozac and the violent murders that had taken place could not be proved beyond a doubt. They also pointed out that thousands of other people were currently taking Prozac with no ill effects, and rather, had been doing well on the drug.

It's interesting to note, however, that the Prozac people used the very same defense favored by the major tobacco companies for many years. For decades, doctors had been warning the public that tobacco caused cancer. The tobacco companies consistently countered with the response that the connection between cancer and tobacco was merely circumstantial evidence, and that no exact medical proof had ever been delivered to make a solid link. It was a brilliant position to take. That's because of the nature of science and the scientific method. Science is an extremely rigorous and exacting discipline, and pinning just about anything down as "definite" and "proven" is actually quite rare in science. However, after a large bodies of evidence are collected and all the facts put together, there comes a point when very good and reliable conclusions can be made, and safely assumed to be "fact." Such is the case with the link between cancer and tobacco. Today, even the major tobacco producers now admit -- finally! -- that their products cause cancer. But now they have simply switched to a different strategy. Today, tobacco company policy is to not deny that their products as addictive and kill people, but rather make the case that people are warned about the risks on every pack of cigarettes that they buy, and it's up to them to choose to smoke or not to smoke.

The Prozac industry is still in the denial phase and they probably have a much better case. Proving that Prozac can actually cause people to kill themselves or others is probably next to impossible. They have a perfect circular kind of defense. For example, a person will only take Prozac if they are already depressed or have some other mental problem. If the person after taking Prozac flies of the handle and kills himself or another person, the Prozac people can say: "Well, he had a problem in the first place. Why else would he be taking Prozac if he wasn't mentally ill!"

So the big drug companies very effectively buried the possibility in the minds of the public that Prozac could turn people into homicidal maniacs, or suicidal nut-cases. The case has never been proven one way or the other. Certainly, even if Prozac does cause some people to become dangerously violent, say less than a half of one percent, that's considered an "acceptable risk" by most standards.

The problem with the latter argument is, however, that millions of prescriptions of Prozac are handed out each year. If only if one-half of one percent of one million people go berserk on Prozac, that means 500 people will potentially kill someone or someone else.

And despite Eli Lilly's -- the manufacturer of Prozac -- attempts to minimize or play down the potential dangers of their "clean drug, the disturbing reports and studies have kept surfacing over the decades.

For example, an article called "The Dangers of fluoxetine" appeared in the January 18, 1997 issue of the highly respected British journal of medicine, Lancet. In the article written by Dr. Robert Bourguignon, of Belgium, he tells of a letter he sent to 500 Belgium physicians asking for reports of serious side effects from Prozac.

The answers he received were very troublesome. Dr. Bourguignon said that eleven doctors reported what he classified as serious events. The side effects which were reported included "a feeling of going to die" and panic attacks; "great nervousness" during just the first 2 weeks of treatment. Other doctors reported "aggressive behavior when Prozac was coupled with alcohol abuse in one patient. Some of the 500 doctors reported "suicidal ideas leading to "paranoid psychosis." In two cases, doctors reported patients on Prozac had nervous breakdowns leading to "barely controllable suicide attempts." Two cases of convulsions were also reported.

Of course, Eli Lilly disputed Dr. Bourguignon's report. They issued a statement which questioned the way the study was done, calling it unscientific, and also restated its belief that Prozac was a safe medication. Dr. Bourguignon said: "The company's reassurance about Prozac's safety of use and efficiency causes some practitioners not to monitor their depressive patients closely enough. Eli Lilly's denial of the existence of these side-effects and refusal to discuss them gives cause for concern. "

But even if we discount the serious potential side effects of Prozac -- suicidal behavior, violent reactions and more -- there is still much more to be concerned about when it comes to the miracle "clean drug" of the century, as some have called it.

When Prozac was first introduced, Eli Lilly made the claim publicly that the drug was "mostly free of side effects." The FDA itself objected to this statement, pointing out that Eli Lilly's own studies showed that some 15% of patients had to discontinue use of the drug due to adverse side effects -- in fact, this information is included on the product label itself!

The fact is, Prozac was shown not to be "mostly free of side effects," but rather had been linked to no less than 242 side effects -- 34 of which included problem with the sexual organs and/or urinary tract of people who took Prozac. Furthermore, according to medical journalist and long-time drug industry critic Thomas J. Moore, Prozac caused more cased of hospitalization over a 10-year period than any other drug in America!

Many other more subtle, but just as disturbing problems are cropping in the media every day. Those who take Prozac regularly report that:

- "It cured my feelings of depression, but the trouble is, it cured ALL of my feelings. Now I don't get sad anymore, but I never feel really happy either. I feel black, like an empty shell."

- "I was no longer depressed on Prozac, but it ended my sex life. I just lost all interest in sex. I'm not sure what to do -- quit Prozac and feel depressed, but have great sex, or continue on Prozac, feel okay, and give up on sex."

- "Prozac made me feel jittery and overly excited all the time. It was great when I wanted to get a lot of work done at the office, but then I could never come down again, like when I wanted a peaceful weekend and home with my family."

- Prozac chased away my blues, but also my ability to have an orgasm. I have never experienced orgasm once since starting Prozac."

Many people who decide to quit Prozac find out that "just stopping" is not all that easy. Thousands of people have reported mild convulsions, and many have reported feelings of electricity shooting through their bodies. Others report feeling more depressed than ever before -- and thus are faced with staying on Prozac for life with all its side effects -- or hoping for some other treatment to come along.

Finally, before we close this chapter and our closer look at the latest "miracle drug" Prozac, it is revealing to take a brief look at the company that makes it. Eli Lilly, and examine the way they operate. As we have said elsewhere in this book, the big drug companies are extremely motivated by the profit motive. The major drug companies like to point out that developing a new drug that could cure or help millions of sick people is a very risky and expensive venture, and they're correct. It takes an average of $500 million dollars to research, develop and test a new drug and finally bring it to market. Then it costs millions more to advertise it, market it, manufacture it and distribute it. Because of this, they claim, they are justified in not only charging enormous prices for each drug, but in doing everything they can to protect its investment.

While this is true, a look at the larger picture reveals some disturbing trends. Drug companies are allowed to keep their patents on a drug they develop for 10 years. After that, they are required to release their patent rights, allowing other drug manufacturers to issue the very same drug as a "generic," greatly reducing the price of the drug to the sick people who need it.

But Eli Lilly fought tooth and nail to get around these federal regulations. For Eli Lilly, Prozac was one of the biggest profit bonanzas in all of prescription drug history. In just a few short years, they recaptured all of their research and development costs, and at a certain point, every dollar they made on Prozac was pure profit. Yet Eli Lilly recently sued for the right to keep Prozac from going generic. They lost the case in the courts. This did not stop Eli Lilly. They then attempted to re-release a different form of Prozac under a different name, and recapture exclusive profits for another 10 years.

Even though the profits from Prozac alone dwarfed the income of whole other industries combined, Eli Lilly did everything it could to make sure their "miracle drug" would cost the average person on the street as much as possible for as long as possible. Clearly, Eli Lilly's major concern is with making money and profits. With such an attitude, can we trust anything they say about the overall safety of the drugs they produce, including their all-time star -- Prozac? Where there's billions of dollars to be made, you can bet there's a lot of people willing to bend the rules, cover up any uncomfortable facts and shape public opinion in a way that ensures those profits will keep flowing -- no matter who dies, who gets hurt, who has his life ruined, or who goes crazy taking a drug they believed would help them have a better life.

EPILOGUE

Just as this book was going to press, the following information was run in a variety of stories over most major media outlets about the drug Paxil, a close cousin of Prozac. Paxil, like Prozac, is a serotonin re-uptake inhibitor.

A lawsuit contends the manufacturer of the popular anti-depressant Paxil concealed evidence that the drug can be addictive. The lawsuit was filed on behalf of 35 people from around the country who say they suffered symptoms ranging from electrical shocks to suicidal thoughts after discontinuing use of the drug. The lawsuit, which seeks class-action status and unspecified damages, says GlaxoSmithkline PLC concealed the possibility of physical and psychological withdrawal symptoms from the drug. It alleges fraud, deceit, negligence, liability, and breach of warranty. The British company has made no comment on the lawsuit. Paxil is the second largest selling anti-depressant in America. In June of 2001, a jury in Wyoming awarded $8 million in damages to a family of a man after determining that Paxil caused him to kill his wife, daughter, and granddaughter before he committed suicide.

-- Source: Associated Press

Chapter Three

There is a national epidemic sweeping America. It's not a dread new disease -- although some consider it that -- but rather a condition. It's obesity. Today, more than ever, people are getting fat, and they're getting fat by the millions. Even children are getting fat. Many people are dangerously overweight by the time they are 10 years old. Some start much earlier than that. Once they get heavy, they spend the rest of their lives battling the bulge -- a battle more often lost than won.

The "experts" blame the new American lifestyle. Today, more people have sit down jobs that require little physical excursion beyond tapping away on a keyboard. It's the same for kids. In years past, kids played baseball, rode their bicycles or ran around with their favorite dog. But today, kids are much more likely to be sitting in front of a computer playing video games, or watching television. While they do so, they are loading up on unhealthy foods. Also among children, the intake of sugary soft drinks is at an all time high. These days a high school student is much more likely to get a Coke from the pop machine in the school hallway than drink milk provided by the school lunch program, or the parent.

All this fat is causing further problems. Being overweight is more than just a cosmetic problem. Obesity leads to all manner of illnesses, but especially diabetes. The amount of people contracted diabetes today it truly astounding. Doctors are calling it a national epidemic. They blame excess weight as the primary culprit. Even a person five to 10 pounds overweight has many times the likelihood of developing diabetes than a person at an optimal weight. Three other major killer are also associated with obesity: Cancer, high blood pressure and heart disease.

Even though obesity is primarily a health care concern, millions of people worry far more about their looks than they do the physical drawbacks of being fat. Women especially are conditioned by society and driven to be as thin as possible. The social pressure to be thin is enormous. Only the "popular" people are thin. Fat people get picked on. On thousands of magazine covers, TV shows and movies, we see mostly beautiful people living exciting lives of passion and adventure. Models for clothing almost never feature an obese person, unless it's a specialty shop catering to "big and tall" folks. A popular buzz terms for overweight people these days is "plus-size" people. But fat is fat, no matter what you call it.

Enter the big drug companies. Realizing that there is a national obsession with getting thin -- while at the same time millions of people are getting fat - the drug companies have smelled huge profits in "magic pills" that can make people thin without all that bothersome stuff, such as exercise, a healthy diet and self discipline. And once again, the drug companies have unleashed a battery of drugs, pills and potions that partially help the problem -- but create even more problems in its wake.

The number of people who have died, or been terribly sickened by diet drugs, both prescription and nonprescription undoubtedly numbers in the hundreds of thousands in America alone.

Perhaps the best example of an extremely dangerous diet drug is the now infamous combination of two different drugs called "fen-phen." The "fen" in fen-phen refers to Pondimin (fenfluramine) and Redux (dexfenfluramine), both sold by the American drug company Wyeth-Ayert Laboratories. We'll talk about a variety of other dangerous diet drugs, both prescription and over-the-counter a bit later, but for now, the story of fen-phen will demonstrate not only the dangers of a specific diet drug, but also the the duplicity and double-dealing of a major drug company.

FEN-PHEN THE FAT KILLER -- THE HUMAN KILLER

In case you have not heard of the prescription diet drug commonly known as fen-phen, the drug refers to the use in combination of fenfluramine and phentermine. The drugs used in combination were approved by the FDA many years ago as appetite suppressants for the short-term weight loss. Phentermine was approved in 1959 and fenfluramine in 1973.

But the combination of the two drugs, called fen-phen, was

approved by the FDA in 1996 for use as an appetite suppressant. After this, many thousands of prescription were handed out by doctors, mostly to women, although some men tried the latest "miracle drug" too. Six million people in the United States took fen-phen.

But just a year later, in 1997, the Mayo Clinic in Minnesota reported that 24 patients had developed heart valve disease after taking fen-phen. In five patients who underwent valve replacement surgery, the diseased valves were found to have distinctive features similar to those seen in carcinoid syndrome. The cluster of unusual cases of valve disease in fen-phen users suggested that there might be an association between fen-phen use and valve disease.

Shortly after, the FDA issued a Public Health Advisory based on the Mayo findings. The Mayo findings were reported in the August 28 issue of the New England Journal of Medicine, along with an FDA letter to the editor describing additional cases. Soon after, the FDA received more than 100 reports of heart valve disease associated mainly with fen-phen. There were also reports of cases of heart valve disease in patients taking only fenfluramine or dexfenfluramine. No cases meeting FDA's definition of a case were reported in patients taking phentermine alone.

At first, there wasn't too much worry because all of the above cases occurred with people who had already had heart disease before they started fen-phen. But then the FDA received reports from five physicians who had performed heart studies on patients who had received fen-phen or dexfen-phen and did not have symptoms of heart disease. Of 291 asymptomatic patients screened, about 30 percent had abnormal valve findings, primarily aortic regurgitation. Based on these data, the drug company, Wyeth-Ayert Laboratories, agreed to withdraw the products from the market and FDA has recommended that patients stop taking the drugs.

In 1992, a number of articles were published about study

results suggesting that the combined use of phentermine and fenfluramine would result in significant weight loss when used over an extended period of time. The results of these studies were not reviewed by FDA, and the conclusion about long-term use of the combination of drugs had never received not received FDA approval.

As it turns out, the people who took fen-phen had changes in their heart valves that caused leakiness and back flow of blood. If this condition gets severe, the heart has to work harder. This may cause problems in heart function. Unfortunately, the patient may have no symptoms. A doctor might hear a new heart murmur when he listens to a heart with a stethoscope, or runs an echocardiogram. If the disease is severe, the patient may experience such symptoms as shortness of breath, excessive tiredness, chest pain, fainting, and swelling of the legs (edema).

It is still unknown if the damage done by fen-phen is reversible. Much seems to depend on the degree of damage. Medications may help the heart function. If the damage is severe, the valves may have to be replaced surgically.

Another problem with fen-phen is that it may interact dangerously with our old friends Prozac, Zoloft and Paxil. This is especially bad since many people who are obese tend also to be depressed. Thus, many people taking fen-phen may also have been prescribed Prozac, vastly increasing the dangers in ways that are unknown.

The end result is that fen-phen killed some people, and gave heart damage to many more. But if you think this is the worst part of the story, you haven't heard the rest.

That's because the maker of fen-phen allegedly paid off a number of prestigious medical journals -- the same respected medical publications whose job it is to keep us all safe -- so that they would write and publish favorable articles about the deadly diet drug. A total of 10 articles were paid for, although only two were published. The other eight might have made it to print, but investigative journalist were getting nosy, and the remaining eight articles favorable to fen-phen, and downplaying its potential side effects were canned.

A drug company spokesman defended the articles. He told a Texas newspaper about the articles:

"This is a common practice in the industry. It's not particular to us," Wyeth spokesman Doug Petkus said. "The companies have some input, it seems, in the initial development of the piece ... but the proposed author has the last say."

But many cried foul. For example, medical ethicists and editors of prominent medical journals criticized the practice as wrong and deceitful. Dr. Robert M. Tenery Jr., chairman of the American Medical Association's council on ethical and judicial affairs said:

"What they're doing here is clearly an advertisement, but it's couched in a scientifically valid paper. ... Some physicians will read this and have no idea that it's not."

And Dr. Jerome P. Kassirer, editor of the New England Journal of Medicine, called Wyeth's conduct "appalling." He said:

"The whole process strikes me as egregious -- the fact that Wyeth commissioned someone to write pieces that are favorable to them, the fact that they paid people to put their names on these things, the fact that people were willing to put their names on it, the fact that the journals published them without asking questions."

So here we see one of the most sorry, deceitful and sad tales in all of U.S. [prescription drug history. A dangerous drug which killed innocent people, and a drug maker that "worked the system" to hide the potential dangers of the drug, and did everything it could to keep the drug on the market and maximize its profits.

ONLY ONE OF MANY

The story of fen-phen, bad as it is, represents just one of the deadly diet drugs. Even though fen-phen is off the market, dieters still should not relax. That's because there are still a number of extremely dangerous diet pill products on the market, and worse yet, most of them are available without a doctor's prescription! That's right. You can walk into drug store or health food store and get a bottle of deadly diet pills, and you may never find out how harmful they truly are. Some people will get lucky and have no ill effects, but others will die before they found out what killed them.

Some of the major diet drug killers on the market today are those that contain an herbal substance called ephedra. Ephedrine alkaloids in dietary supplements are usually derived from one of several species of herbs of the genus Ephedra, sometimes called Ma huang, Chinese Ephedra and epitonin. Other botanical sources include Sida cordifolia. Ephedrine alkaloids, as they are known, are amphetamine-like compounds with potentially powerful stimulant effects on the nervous system and heart. Hundreds of consumer illnesses and injuries associated with the use of these products have been reported. Because ephedrine alkaloids are heart and nervous system stimulants, some people, especially those with high blood pressure, heart conditions and neurologic disorders are playing it dangerously when they use such products. Pregnant women, too, should avoid the use of dietary supplements with ephedrine alkaloids.

Despite their dangers, the FDA has not moved to ban such products, even they are aware that people have died from them. Instead, they have published a series of "safety guidelines" for people who still want to play with this deadly stuff.

The FDA has also proposed that dietary supplements containing ephedrine alkaloids should have limits on the amount of the stuff contained in products. They also suggest a warning label and other "marketing measures" to give adequate warning and information to consumers.

The FDA proposal would also prohibit the marketing of dietary supplements containing 8 milligrams or more of ephedrine alkaloids per serving. Labeling that recommends or suggests conditions of use that would result in an intake of 8 mg or more in a 6-hour period or a total daily intake of 24 mg or more also would not be allowed. Also, the proposal would require label statements instructing consumers not to use the product for more than 7 days, and would not allow label claims for uses for which long-term intake would be necessary to achieve the purported effect. These safety measures are based on the fact that long-term intake of ephedrine alkaloids increases the likelihood of serious adverse events.

Still further, the FDA would require instructions on the products claims that would encourage short-term excessive intake to enhance the claimed effect, such as energy enhancement. They want the products to bear a labeling statement saying that "Taking more than the recommended serving may result in heart attack, stroke, seizure or death."

The FDA proposal also would prohibit the use of other stimulant ingredients such as botanical sources of caffeine with ephedrine alkaloids because the combination increases the stimulant effects of ephedrine alkaloids and the chance of consumer injury.

The FDA proposed all these changes because they received and investigated more than 800 reports of adverse events associated with the use of these products. Reported adverse events range from episodes of high blood pressure, irregularities in heart rate, insomnia, nervousness, tremors and headaches, to seizures, heart attacks, strokes and death. Most events occurred in young to middle aged, otherwise healthy adults using the products for weight control and increased energy.

And still they decided not to ban it! Do you still want to take a dietary supplement containing ephedra? It's your choice. It's okay with the FDA. You make the decision!

In the meantime, here are some other diet supplements the FDA has issued warnings about:

• **Comfrey** (Symphytum officionale (common comfrey), Sasperum (prickley comfrey), and S. x uplandicum (Russian comfrey).

These plants are a source of pyrrolizidine alkaloids that present a serious health hazard to consumers when they are ingested. The use of comfrey in dietary supplements is a serious concern to FDA, they say. These plants contain pyrrolizidine alkaloids, substances which are firmly established to be hepatotoxins in animals. Reports in the scientific literature clearly associate oral exposure of comfrey and pyrrolizidine alkaloids with the occurrence of veno-occlusive disease (VOD) in animals. Moreover, outbreaks of hepatic VOD have been reported in other countries over the years and the toxicity of these substances in humans is generally accepted. The use of products containing comfrey has also been implicated in serious adverse incidents over the years in the United States and elsewhere.

The adverse effects that have been seen with comfrey are entirely consistent with the known effects of comfrey ingestion that have been described in the scientific literature. The pyrrolizidine alkaloids that are present in comfrey, in addition to being potent hepatotoxins, have also been shown to be toxic to other tissues as well. There is also evidence that implicates these substances as carcinogens. Taken together, the clear evidence of an association between oral exposure to pyrrolizidine alkaloids and serious adverse health effects and the lack of any valid scientific data that would enable the agency to determine whether there is an exposure, if any, that would present no harm to consumers, indicates that this substance should not be used as an ingredient in dietary supplements.

ANOTHER DANGER DIET DRUG -- TRIAC

Dietary supplements that contain tiratricol, also known as triiodothyroacetic acid or TRIAC, a potent thyroid hormone that may cause serious health consequences including heart attacks and strokes. Despite four recalls over the past seven months, various products that contain tiratricol may still have reached consumers. FDA urges all consumers to stop using such products immediately.

On November 11, 1999, FDA warned the public against consuming Triax Metabolic Accelerator, a dietary supplement for weight loss by Syntrax Innovations, Inc., Cape Giradeau, Mo. Since this action, several other firms have recalled similar products containing tiratricol. Distribution of these products has been primarily through retail sales to health food stores, fitness centers, and gymnasiums.

Please note: In the chapter in this book you will find important information on a number of other herbal and natural dietary supplements that have been deemed to be possibly very dangerous. We urge you to read that chapter and learn the facts before you choose to buy any diet products whatsoever.

Conclusions

The story of diet drugs is very sad indeed. Whether it be a deceitful and greedy major drug producer putting a deadly product in the hands of doctors, or dozens of so-called "health food" providers making all manner of dangerous herbal diet remedies, the story is always the same --people who are looking for an "easy" magic pill" remedy for a condition that is best not treated with drugs at all. What is the best way to lose weight? It's no secret. You eat less and exercise more! You also eat foods that will not make you fat, while favoring low-fat healthy food that will energize your body without starving it. Once again, the people of America must stop trusting pill makers, and start trusting themselves. They must take their own lives and their own problems into their own hands and do something about them sensibly. A pill most often do nothing for you -- except sicken or kill you.

Chapter Four

Accutane -- Suicide, Cancer and Deformed Babies in the Name of Clear Skin

For years, teenagers everywhere have suffered through the heartbreak of faces peppered with acne. Just before that first date, or on prom night, those ugly zits have a way of popping up on the face like mushrooms across a cow pasture. But for many teens, the problem is more than just the occasional pimple. Thousands of teens suffer from an entire face, chest, back, throat and other parts of the body covered with angry red welts that leak, bleed, and worst of all, look hideous. The result, especially for the delicate, highly self conscious mind of today's young people goes well beyond physical pain. The psychological results can be devastating. They are shunned by their peers, or worse, taunted and excluded from cohorts and camaraderie.

It's a golden opportunity for the major drug companies to come up with a solution -- and perhaps more importantly to them --

a lot of profits.

Enter the drug Accutane, known generically as isotretinoin. Accutane is a drug used to treat the most severe form of acne (nodular acne) that cannot be cleared up by any other acne treatments, including antibiotics. In severe nodular acne, many red, swollen, tender lumps form in the skin. These can be the size of pencil erasers or larger. If untreated, nodular acne can lead to permanent scars.

The new drug Accutane seemed another pharmaceutical miracle. It has proved extremely effective in clearing up skin, and the fact that it is not an antibiotic made doctors more willing to prescribe it. Even so, doctors and medical researchers are not sure just how this drug works. They know it DOES work, but the exact why of it is still a mystery. Accutane reduces the amount of sebum in the skin. Sebum is a natural oily skin lubricant. It shrinks the glands that produce sebum. It also inhibits what is called keratinization, which is hardening of the skin cells.

Once Accutane was introduced onto the market, teenagers lined up by the thousand to rid themselves of the long hated scourge of acne. Suddenly young faces all over America were clear and bright. Medical science seemed to have done it again. Accutane was lauded by the media and medical doctors as a great victory over a skin disease that has caused a million heartaches, and permanent acne scarring over countless years.

But then, like so many other miracle drugs, a darker underside of Accutane began to make itself known. Suddenly, once normal and happy teenagers began to have frightening changes in personality. Many grew morbidly depressed. Many inexplicably committed suicide. Still others grew violent and turned to criminal behavior. Many of these once normal teens all had one thing in common -- they all had experienced bad acne, and they all had treated it with a prescription of Accutane.

Then, even more problems began to emerge. Many young women who had taken Accutane, or who were currently taking Accutane, began to bear deformed babies, or babies born dead. Could it have been the drug Accutane that had cause the problem? In fact, Accutane soon began to be recognized by doctors as the most potent birth defect producer since the 1950s, when the drug thalidomide caused thousands of babies to be born hideously deformed. Accutane has caused babies to be born with grossly enlarged skulls, with undersized or absent ears, with misshapen eyes, cleft palates, and distorted faces. Other babies were born with malfunctioning thyroid or thymus glands. Even when a baby looks normal physically, babies born with Accutane effects often have IQs of less than 85. Accutane may also produce bone marrow damage in infants.

If all of the above is not bad enough, Accutane also has serious links to cancer. In lab experiments, rats developed cancer after just 18 months on Accutane. The studies on rat strongly suggested that Accutane could disturb the most fundamental building block of the human body -- DNA. In the rats that did not develop cancer, a number of other serious health problems developed., including inflammation of the heart, fibrous growths, calcification of the heart vessels and other blood vessels, and clouded eye corneas.

But the book on Accutane side effects is still not closed. It is now believed that the drug can disrupt the basic cell division in any part of the human body. Because of this, and because of the well known affect on bone marrow, Accutane may be responsible for many thousands of deaths. The exact number may never be known. But because Accutane is distributed to millions of people per year, there can be little doubt that the death rate will continue to be high, and may never be fully known.

Because of all these serious problems, the Dermatologic and

Ophthalmic Drugs Advisory Committee on September 18 and 19, 2000, concluded that further steps are necessary in addition to the warnings already in place by the manufacturer and the FDA to ensure the safe use of this drug. The Committee recommended:

1. Developing limitations on the appropriate use of the drug:

Additional systematized measures to manage risk and fully inform patients and families should be instituted, given the devastating impact o potential side effects.

2. Educational efforts to prevent pregnancy exposure:

Despite the effort of the makers of Accutane's to educate the public on the dangers of birth defects, a significant proportion of fetal exposures has still occurred because patients were already pregnant at the time of starting Accutane. These events are entirely preventable. It is well known in the field of safety that exclusive reliance on "human memory" is not an adequate precaution for managing severe risks. Systems approaches, which build in mandated safety checks at critical points, provide much more effective support for prescribers, dispensers, and patients.

3. Psychiatric Events:

With respect to psychiatric events, the committee agreed that no clear causal link has been established. However, definitive demonstration of causality for a rare adverse event can be difficult to demonstrate. When there is reasonable suspicion of an association, patients should be informed. More scientific study of this issue in still needed but it must be recognized that the design of informative trials presents significant methodologic and ethical challenges.

WHAT YOU SHOULD KNOW AND DO ABOUT ACCUTANE0

FOR WOMEN:

Women must realize that Accutane can cause birth defects if taken by a pregnant woman. It can also cause miscarriage, premature birth, or death of the baby. Do not take Accutane if you are pregnant or plan to become pregnant while you are taking Accutane, or for 1 month after you stop taking Accutane. Also, if you get pregnant while taking Accutane, stop taking it right away and call your doctor.

Women must not become pregnant while taking Accutane, or for 1 month after you stop taking Accutane. Accutane can cause severe birth defects in babies of women who take it while they are pregnant, even if they take Accutane for only a short time. There is an extremely high risk that your baby will be deformed or will die if you are pregnant while taking Accutane. Taking Accutane also increases the chance of losing the baby before it is born (miscarriage) and early (premature) births.

Female patients cannot get their first prescription for Accutane unless there is proof from 2 tests that they are not pregnant. One test must be done on one of these 2 dates, whichever is later: the second day of your next period 11 days after you last had sexual intercourse without using birth control Women can get a prescription for Accutane only when the required testing shows you are not pregnant. Female patients cannot get monthly refills for Accutane, unless there is proof that they are not pregnant.

While women are taking Accutane, you must use effective birth control. You must use 2 separate effective forms of birth control at the same time for at least 1 month before starting Accutane, while you take it, and for 1 month after you stop taking it. You can either discuss effective birth control methods with your provider or go for a free visit to discuss birth control with someone else. Your doctor can arrange this free visit.

Women must use 2 separate forms of effective birth control because any method, including birth control pills and sterilization, can fail. Further, no one knows if Accutane lowers the effectiveness of birth control pills or injections (shots). There are only 2 reasons you would not need to use 2 separate methods of effective birth control:

You have had your uterus removed by surgery (hysterectomy). You commit to complete abstinence. This means that you are absolutely positive that you will not have genital-to-genital sexual contact before, during, and for 1 month after Accutane treatment. If you have sex without using effective birth control or miss your period, stop using Accutane and call your doctor right away.

ACCUTANE AND MENTAL PROBLEMS

Some patients, while taking Accutane or soon after stopping Accutane, have become depressed or developed other serious mental problems. Signs of these problems include feelings of sadness, irritability, unusual tiredness, trouble concentrating, and loss of appetite. Some patients taking Accutane have had thoughts about hurting themselves or putting an end to their own lives (suicidal thoughts). Some people tried to end their own lives. And some people have ended their own lives. There were reports that some of these people did not appear depressed. No one knows if Accutane caused these behaviors or if they would have happened even if the person did not take Accutane.

What are the signs of mental problems? Here are some guidelines:

Tell your doctor if, to the best of your knowledge, you or someone in your family has ever had any mental illness, including depression, suicidal behavior, or psychosis. Psychosis means a loss of contact with reality, such as hearing voices or seeing things that are not there. Also, tell your doctor if you take medicines for any of these problems.

Stop using Accutane and tell your provider right away if you:

- Start to feel sad or have crying spells
- Lose interest in your usual activities
- Have changes in your normal sleep patterns
- Become more irritable than usual
- Lose your appetite
- Become unusually tired
- Have trouble concentrating
- Withdraw from family and friends
- Start having thoughts about hurting yourself/myself or taking your/my own life (suicidall thoughts)

IF YOU STILL WANT TO TAKE ACCUTANE:

Your doctor will give you a 1 month supply of Accutane at a time. This is to make sure you check in with your provider each month to discuss side effects. Your doctor will determine the amount of Accutane you should take. This means is is very risky to make any changes on your own, and without informing your doctor that you are doing so. Most people will take Accutane 2 times a day with food, unless a doctor advises otherwise. f you miss a dose, just skip that dose. Do not take 2 doses the next time. You should return to your provider as directed to make sure you don't have signs of serious side effects. Because some of Accutane's serious side effects show up in blood tests, some of these visits may involve blood tests.

WHAT TO AVOID WHILE TAKING ACCUTANE

Do not get pregnant while taking Accutane. Do not breast feed while taking Accutane and for 1 month after stopping Accutane. It is not known if Accutane can pass through human milk and harm human baby.

Do not give blood while you take Accutane and for 1 month after stopping Accutane. If someone who is pregnant gets your donated blood, her baby may be exposed to Accutane and may be born with birth defects.

Do not take Vitamin A supplements. Vitamin A in high doses has many of the same side effects as Accutane. Taking both together may increase your chance of getting side effects.

Do not have cosmetic procedures to smooth your skin, including waxing, dermabrasion, or laser procedures, while you are using Accutane and for at least 6 months after you stop. Accutane can increase your chance of scarring from these procedures. Check with your provider for advice about when you can have cosmetic procedures.

Avoid sunlight and ultraviolet lights as much as possible. Tanning machines use ultraviolet lights. Accutane may make your skin more sensitive to light.

Do not use birth control pills that have a low dose of progesterone (minipills). They may not work while you take Accutane.

Do not share Accutane with other people. It can cause birth defects and other serious health problems.

Do not take antibiotics with Accutane unless you talk to your doctor. For some antibiotics, you may have to stop taking Accutane until the antibiotic treatment is finished. Use of both drugs together can increase the chances of getting increased pressure in the brain.

A SUMMARY OF SIDE EFFECTS OF ACCUTANE TO WATCH FOR

• Accutane can cause birth defects, premature births, and death in babies whose mothers took Accutane while they were pregnant.

• Serious mental health problems. (See above).

• Serious brain problems. Accutane can increase the pressure in your brain. This can lead to permanent loss of sight, or in rare cases, death. Stop taking Accutane and call your doctor right away if you get any of these signs of increased brain pressure: bad headache, blurred vision, dizziness, nausea, or vomiting.

• Some patients taking Accutane have had seizures (convulsions) or stroke.

• Abdomen (stomach area) problems. Certain symptoms may mean that your internal organs are being damaged. These organs include the liver, pancreas, and bowel (intestines). If your organs are damaged, they may not get better even after you stop taking Accutane. Stop taking Accutane and call your provider if you get severe stomach or bowel pain, diarrhea, rectal bleeding, yellowing of your skin or eyes, or dark urine.

• Bone and muscle problems. Accutane may affect bones, muscles, and ligaments and cause pain in your joints or muscles. Tell your provider if you plan vigorous physical activity during treatment with Accutane. Tell your doctor if you develop pain. If a bone breaks, tell your provider you take Accutane. No one knows if taking Accutane for acne will reduce bone healing or stunt growth.

• Hearing problems. Some people taking Accutane have developed hearing problems. It is possible that hearing loss can be permanent. Stop using Accutane and call your provider if your hearing gets worse or if you have
ringing in your ears.

• Vision problems. While taking Accutane you may develop a

sudden inability to see in the dark, so driving at night can be dangerous. This condition usually clears up after you stop taking Accutane, but it may be permanent. Other serious eye effects can occur. Stop taking Accutane and call your provider right away if you have any problems with your vision or dryness of the eyes that is painful or constant.

• Lipid (fats and cholesterol in blood) problems. Many people taking Accutane develop high levels of cholesterol and other fats in their blood. This can be a serious problem. Return to your doctor for blood tests to check your lipids and to get any needed treatment. These problems generally go away when Accutane treatment is finished.

• Allergic reactions. In some people, Accutane can cause serious allergic reactions. Stop taking Accutane and get emergency care right away if you develop hives, a swollen face or mouth, or have trouble breathing. Stop taking Accutane and call your provider if you develop a fever, rash, or red patches or bruises on your legs.

• Breathing problems. Tell your doctor if you have trouble breathing (shortness of breath), are fainting, are very thirsty or urinate a lot, feel weak, have leg swelling, convulsions, slurred speech, problems moving, or any other serious or unusual problems. Frequent urination and thirst can be signs of blood sugar problems.

It should be noted that serious permanent problems do not happen often, but if they happen to you, that's small comfort. Because the symptoms listed above may be signs of serious problems, if you get them, stop taking Accutane and call your provider. If not treated, they could lead to serious health problems. Even if these problems are treated, they may not clear up after you stop taking Accutane.

SOME LESS SERIOUS PROBLEMS

The common less serious side effects of Accutane are dry

skin, chapped lips, dry eyes, and dry nose that may lead to nosebleeds. People who wear contact lenses may have trouble wearing them while taking Accutane and after therapy. Sometimes, people's acne may get worse for a while. They should continue taking Accutane unless told to stop by their doctor.

But please remember that all we have listed here are definitely not all of Accutane's possible side effects. Your doctor or pharmacist can give you more detailed information that is written for health care professionals.

What we have provided here is only a summary of some important information about Accutane. Medicines are sometimes prescribed for purposes other than those listed in a Medication Guide. If you have any concerns or questions about Accutane, ask your doctor. Do not use Accutane for a condition for which it was not prescribed.

Conclusions

Accutane is yet another sad story about a drug sold to the general public as safe, only to discover after many deaths, birth defects and severely sickened people. With the release of Accutane, millions of young people saw hope for an end to the psychologically debilitating disease of severe acne. Why did the FDA approve this drug for use among the general public? Was its approval process flawed? Did they get pressure from the drug companies to rush Accutane through the process? Did the makers of Accutane donate money to the campaign funds of key Congressmen to help the drug get through the system faster? These are all serious questions that deserve answers.

And finally this: Although severe acne is no laughing matter and a disease that deserves serious treatment, it is not a life threatening disease, and more a matter of psychological and cosmetic concern. Today, our society puts a huge emphasis on looks, appearance and beauty. Young people and teenagers are especially concerned with how they look, being popular and attractive to the opposite sex. But in this case, we can certainly state that this particular problem is truly skin deep. The vast majority of teen acne cases clear up without the need for drugs as the person matures and enters his or her twenties. By then, those old days of acne are forgotten and life goes on as normal. We must all ask ourselves, is a clear face and a pretty complexion worth dying for? Is it worth unleashing a drug as deadly and as rife with problems as is Accutane? Once again, we see the overwhelming public attitude that just about anything and everything can be "cured" by simply taking a "magic pill." There are a lot of profit hungry drug manufacturers ready and willing to exploit this attitude in exchange for enormous sums of money. The fact that people will be killed, sickened, or born with horrible life-long birth defects seems almost beside the point.

Until the public adjusts its expectations and attitudes toward powerful prescription drugs, and an all too willingness to experiment with them, there will always be another Accutane, another Prozac, another Baycol waiting in the wings to take more lives or sicken more people.

LATE BREAKING ACCUTANE NEWS

Just as we were going to press with this book, we noticed the following information released in a variety of major media sources:

The US Centers for Disease Control and Prevention (CDC) released a report indicating that some women taking the acne drug Accutane become pregnant despite efforts to warn them that the product is known to cause severe birth defects. Furthermore, the CDC also said that a symbol used to remind women of the birth defect effects of medicines is very often misinterpreted.

The makers of Accutane and doctors recommend that women have two negative pregnancy tests, including one on the second day of their next normal menstrual period, before taking the medication. Also, women taking Accutane should use two forms of birth control, have repeat pregnancy tests every month and register with a survey that monitors the experience of women taking the drug.

The CDC said that more than 2,000 pregnancies in US women taking Accutane were reported to the Food and Drug Administration (FDA) between 1982 and March 2000.

The makers of Accutane, New Jersey-based Roche, told said that they company was not aware of the CDC report, but the problem of birth defects associated with Accutane continues to be "a very critical issue."

Said said Roche,

"This drug has been on the market since September 1982 and ever since we received our first birth defect report shortly thereafter...we have continued to work with not only the (FDA) but the dermatology community to strengthen our warnings."

Roche officials also said they have taken a number of steps to deal with the issue of Accutane-related birth defects, including the strengthening of warnings on labels and the provision of free pregnancy tests and gynecological counseling for patients.

Even so, Roche admits the problem of birth defects and women not seeing them or ignoring them is an ongoing problem. Roche said it will continue to work with the FDA to develop solutions.

One of the major problems with the current warning signs being used on Accutane is that women do not recognize it. The symbol is a pregnant woman depicted in a circle with a slash through it. Many women reported not knowing what this meant or referred to. Many women assumed it had something to do with birth control.

The CDC is now recommending that drug manufacturers and marketers make certain that drug package text and symbols are clear and cannot increase risk to consumers. Also, the CDC said that health providers should make sure that their patients taking drugs that can cause birth defects are fully aware of the risks.

CONCLUSIONS

As we can see from this final news about Accutane, even strenuous and obvious efforts to warn women that the drug may cause birth defects are not 100% effective -- not even close. The drug continues to change lives forever -- it continues to bring babies into the world that are hideously deformed, mentally retarded, or possibly born dead. Yet, this drug is not an essential "life saving" drug. Far from it. It's a drug that merely gives teen a clear face -- something that many of them will have anyway in a few years. Also, there are other, safer drugs, and even nondrug natural ways to deal with acne. Given all of the above, why does not Roche simply take the drug off the market. You will notice all the "PR speak" in the above story about Accutane. The drug's maker, Roche, blandly states that it is "doing everything it can" to prevent further birth defects and that it is "working with the FDA" to resolve the problem. Roche also said it is "concerned."

But apparently not concerned enough to simply pull the drug off the market. That would mean billions in lost sales revenue. Roche feels that a few deformed and dead babies are a small price to pay to bolster their bottom line and keep the faces of teenagers as clean as a glossy fashion magazine.

Chapter Five

THEY DIED TRYING TO LOWER THEIR CHOLESTEROL -- THE DRUG INDUSTRY STRIKES AGAIN

Like millions of average Americans, Bob Preston, age 50, was just slightly overweight, and he loved to eat. His favorite meal was a juicy t-bone steak sizzled over an open grill. Bob was not much for vegetables. He was strictly a meat-and-potatoes kind of guy. In other words, Bob was like a lot of people, or even most people. The trouble is, Bob's meat-heavy diet was coating his veins with a thick fatty build-up of cholesterol. The arteries in his heart were beginning to block, leaving Bob short of breath and with minor chest pains.

Bob went to see his doctor. A blood test revealed a cholesterol level of almost 300 -- way to high! Bob's doctor said he needed to get his cholesterol count below 200. To do that, he'd need to change his diet -- less meat, and more fruits, grains and vegetables. Bob's doctor also told him he needed to exercise more. At this time, Bob's most rigorous activity was pushing the remote control buttons on the remote for his satellite television, which featured more than 150 channels. Bob played the occasional game of golf, but other than that, he was strictly a couch potato.

But Bob's doctor had put the fear of God into him. His doctor told him he was heading for a heart attack, or possible even a stroke if he didn't change his ways Of course, both Bob and his doctor knew that a life-time meat eater was not going to become a vegetarian overnight, and that he was not about to take up jogging or tennis. At first, Bob tried taking regular walks in the evening, but quickly got bored with it. Also, Bob would have had to walk at least four miles a night, while cutting down on fatty foods, to start his high cholesterol level going back down in the right direction.

So, like millions of other high cholesterol patients, Bob was given a prescription of a drug which would do all the hard work for him. The drug the doctor gave him was called Baycol, and it was manufactured by one of the most trusted drug producers in the world --Bayer -- the maker so of Bayer aspirin. Buckley is a cholesterol lowering drug designs to melt away the fat lining the veins and arteries of people, without their having to make radical changes in their diet, or lifestyle. Buckley is in an extremely popular class of drugs called statins, which are indicated for lowering cholesterol.

At first, the Baycol seemed to be doing the job for Bob. After a three months on the drug, he returned to the doctor for a blood test, and the results were dramatic. Bob's cholesterol was way down, near the 200 mark, just about where it should be. In the meantime, Bob thought he had it made. He forgot about eating like a rabbit, and balked at the idea of getting out and walking four miles a night when he could be resting comfortably in his living room in front of the boob tube.

But after another couple of months, Bob began to have strange pains, especially in his legs and lower back. Bob began to experience muscle pain throughout many parts of his body. At the same time, Bob began to feel generally less healthy and sickly. He vomited occasionally, had a persistent low-grade fever and saw that the color of his urine had grown darker. He began to loose his appetite, and the pain in his lower back began to get more intense. Worried, bob made an appointment to see his doctor again -- perhaps another magic pill is what he needed again. But Bob never made it to his next appointment -- he died suddenly in his bed one evening, just two days before he was due back at the clinic for his check-up.

The cause of death was strange and frightening. Bob had died of kidney failure. The cause of his death was listed as rhabdomyolsis -- a somewhat rare and frightening disease in which the muscles cells in the body are destroyed and released into the bloodstream. The result is severe muscle pain, and if it goes far enough, it causes the kidneys to fail because they become poisoned by the dead muscle cells which are carried to the kidneys by the blood.

But what had brought on this dread disease, rhabdomyolsis, in Bob's body. It was most likely the very drug that was supposed to save his life -- Baycol, manufactured by Bayer Pharmaceutical. At the time this book went to press, more than 700,000 Americans were taking Baycol. But in early August of 2001, the U.S. Food and Drug Administration ordered the drug to be pulled from the market because it had been identified with at least 31 deaths in the United States, and at least nine death in foreign countries. The FDA recommends that anyone currently taking Baycol contact their doctor and take immediate action to either stop the drug, or switch to a different medication.

But the problem is, which drug should a patient switch to? Baycol is actually just one of an entire class of popular cholesterol lowering drugs, or statins, which include these major names -- Lipitor, Zocor, Lescol, Mevacor and Pravachol. Even though they all have different names, experts feel the statins are much more alike than
different, though they may differ slightly in potency.All of them have the potential to cause the same muscle destroying action in the human body as, does Baycol, although Baycol seems to be in a class by itself in terms of it's danger. Still, the negative side effect of the other popular statins is now in questions.

While at least 40 deaths have now been confirmed as a result of Baycol, doctors think there may have been hundreds of cases of rhabdomyolsis attacks throughout the world as a result of this drug.

Dr. John Jenkins of the FDA told the Associated Press said he did not know how many Baycol users have survived a rhabdomyolsis attack, but that the problem is a serious one, and more deaths may have occurred. Jenkins said that there is no reason for public panic, but also urged anyone taking Baycol to stop immediately.

Jenkins also said that people taking another cholesterol lowering drug called gemfibrozil should immediately stop Baycol and contact their doctor. The people most at risk from Baycol and gemfibrozil are elderly who use higher doses. In the United States, 12 of the 31 people who died from rhabdomyolsis were taking both drugs at the same time.

Interestingly, Bayer executives have agreed to pull the drug off the market in all countries, except Japan. Their reasoning is that the Baycol dosages sold in that country are smaller than that used in other nations, so that the risk is less. A cynical observer would again shake his or her head in wonder at the incredible willingness of major pharmaceutical companies to put profit over the safety of the very people is is supposed to be serving and helping toward a more healthy existence. After more than 40 documented deaths worldwide, one would think Bayer would pull the drug altogether to avoid any risk what-so-ever, but apparently they think the people of Japan do not have to worry about having their own muscles dissolve inside their own bodies because they are taking smaller doses of this killer drug.

A British doctor, Dr. Sidney Wolfe, is head of a consumer advocacy group called Public Citizen. He is preparing a petition for the FDA to strengthen warnings on all other statin class drugs, including the popular Lipitor, Pravachol, and the others. His group is also drafting a letter to Japanese authorities urging them to pull Baycol from the market in Japan.

Baycol has become the 12th prescription drug to be pulled from the U.S. market because of dangerous side-effects since 1997.

Many critics of the drug industry said the fact that these dangerous drugs made it top market is the fault of the FDA, which sped up its drug approval process under political pressure from politicians who were being heavily lobbied by the wealthy drug manufacturers. Although Baycol was not one of those so-called "fast-track" drugs, the fact that other drugs are getting even less scrutiny than this killer did should not make the public feel any safer.

The sad story of Baycol is yet another example of a prescription drug designed and sold as a life saving and life extending drug which ends up to be just the opposite for many unfortunate individuals. It must be said that drugs like Baycol and others may have saved many lives to in those cases where it worked properly, lowering cholesterol levels and preventing people from having heart attacks.

But perhaps the real moral of this story can be found when go back to the case of Bob Preston. For the record, Bob is not a real person, but an imaginary name we used to illustrate a very real scenario. Many of the real 31 Americans who were taking Baycol, and who died from it, where just like Bob. They were living lifestyles that contributed to their own deaths, long before a prescription drug came along to finish the job much faster. People like Bob have come to believe that they can have it all -- bad habits, poor diets, little or no exercise -- and when their health begins to fall apart, they assume some magical pill given to them by a doctor will fix everything up with no effort at all. This is the classic "magic bullet" mentality. It's the belief that swallowing a pill is the easiest way to perfect good health.

Our friend Bob could be alive today if he would have taken the more difficult, but ultimately more rewarding road of dealing with his high cholesterol through natural means. Bob could have got up off the couch, shut off the TV and started a daily exercise regimen. He could have taken up any one of a number of enjoyable and life-expanding activities -- walking a few miles a day with friends, or with a happy dog. He could have taken up racket ball, or played a rigorous 18 holes of golf every day. Bob also could have taken a more positive view of a diet change. Yes, it's difficult for a died-in-the-wool meat lover to change over to a more fruit and vegetable oriented diet. But Bob would not have had to become a vegetarian -- he simply needed to mix in more greens, grains, and fish into his weekly diet. He could still cheat with a nice juicy steak now and then, and still see his cholesterol level drop steadily downward.

But instead, Bob trusted in the prescription drug industry and died from a horrible condition in which his own muscles dissolved, fowled up his kidneys and killed him. Americans and people everywhere must stop expecting all of their health problems to be fixed without effort and by taking the easy way out. Sometimes there is no alternative to taking a prescription drug, but in those cases where they can clearly be avoided, that is the option people should go for -- and live to to enjoy the healthy choice they have made for themselves. This is probably more true for the widespread problem of high cholesterol than just about any other disease.

THE STATINS -- MIRACLE DRUG OR ANOTHER DEADLY FALSE HOPE?

When the statin, including Baycol, were first released on the market they were given that same "miracle" status so many other drugs were given, only to find later that these new miracles came with some pretty powerful curses -- including death to the user.

For example, the highly respected Dr. Tim Johnson, the medical editor for ABC News talked a bit about their possible dangers, but dismissed them as extremely minor. The ABC News story had this to say about statins:

"Doctors have found that statins are remarkably safe," Johnson said. Indeed, they have been widely used for a number of

years. Patients who are pregnant, have active or chronic liver disease or those allergic to statins shouldn't use statin drugs, according to the American Heart Association. But for those who can use the drugs, only two problems have been seen with them, Johnson said. About 1 percent of patients have experienced problems with liver functions, so when physicians give the drugs, they have to monitor liver function every six months or so, Johnson said. Also, very rarely, doctors have seen myopathy, or muscle inflammation. But that condition goes away when the drug is decreased or eliminated. And both problems are extremely rare and\ reversible, Johnson said. He doesn't believe that everyone should rush out and get the drugs, but he said those who are older and at greater risk for coronary artery disease or stroke, and especially those at risk for high cholesterol, should talk to their doctors about statins.

"The most important thing is that there are so many people who could benefit from these drugs, especially those with high cholesterol and coronary disease who aren't taking them," Johnson said. "These are almost miraculous for that purpose."

THE ABC News Story on statins continues:

And in the past several years, the statins have been shown to help other diseases. From Alzheimer's to Osteoporosis Dr. Tim Johnson told Good Morning America that in recent years these drugs have shown they might help prevent or reduce the risk for strokes, diabetes and other diseases. "We have studies that suggest they strengthen bone and may reduce the risk for osteoporosis. And probably most amazing of all, there are studies that show that they may significantly reduce the risk for Alzheimer's. All of these things have yet to be fully proven, but there are a lot of studies hinting in this," said Johnson.

So here we see all the regular buzz words -- "miracle," "amazing," side effects that are "rare and reversible," and only "1%

of patients" experience liver problems, and so on. It's almost as if the major media outlets were on the payroll of the big drug companies. This ABC News story demonstrates how easy it is for the drug companies to get the media to do its promotion for them. The ABC News story above was perhaps worth more than a million dollars in advertising to the drug companies, but it was dished out to them for free.

Certainly, ABC News cannot be blamed for merely reporting the facts as they knew them at the time. On the other hand, it is the job of such media entities to be extremely skeptical, and to dig deeper into subjects before hauling off to praise newly discovered drugs -- with no real long-term information about them yet available -- as "amazing" and "miracles." Also to be fair, it was ABC News and others that rushed out to report the deadly aspects of statins as soon as they were discovered, Still, by then, more than a 100 people were dead, and possibly hundreds more. The damage had already been done.

When Baycol was revealed as a major killer, news organizations were quick to point out that it was probably the deadliest of all the statins, and that the others were probably much safer. But just a week after this information, more bad news about the statin family arose. As it turns out, at least 81 more deaths were connected to Baycol's sisters -- Mevacor, Pravachol , Zocor, Lescol, and Lipitor.

According to News Services, a consumer protection group called Public Citizen Health Research Group petitioned the FDA to strengthen warnings about statin. Said Dr. Sydney Wolfe of Public Citizen:

"Most people taking these drugs aren't aware that they could sustain serious muscle damage and could even die. Serious muscle and kidney damage, and potentially death, may be averted only if the patients taking statins stop the drugs at the first sign of muscle pain or weakness."

The advocacy group wants statin labels to include black box warnings -- which are reserved for drugs with unusually serious side effects. This would be an elevated warning from the current cautionary information about the risk of rhabdomylosis, the breakdown of muscle tissue that is a rare side effect of statins. The disease initially causes muscle pain and tiredness. In severe cases it can lead to kidney failure and death.

The Public Citizen group also wants drug companies that make statins to be required to send letter to all U.S. doctors warning about the drug's risks. The group also asks that a guide describing the hazards be given to statin consumers.

Other less deadly but still troubling side effects of statins include gastrointestinal, including constipation and abdominal pain and cramps. These symptoms are usually mild to severe and generally subside as therapy continues. However, the longer a person uses statins, the greater the chance of the deadly muscle disease we described above.

Finally, many of the statins have been shown to cause cancer in rats and mice. Even though the rats had been on the drug only two years before they developed cancer, many people are expected to stay on the drug for a chilling 10 years! This greatly increases the chance of not only developing the deadly muscle disease associated with statins, but also possible liver cancer and other forms of cancer.

So now you have the "rest of the story" on yet another drug touted by the big, profit hungry drug companies as the next "miracle" drug. Reading this chapter in this book may very well have just saved your life! If you are currently taking statins, or are considering taking statins, you might be advised to think twice. Especially when you consider that perfectly natural and safe methods of reducing cholesterol already exist, it makes little sense to risk your life by taking these kind of drugs. A simple change of diet and daily exercise may be all you need. Yes, adopting a new diet and taking up exercise seems extremely difficult to most people. It always seems much easier to just swallow a "magic" pill -- but as is always the case with something that seems too good to be true -- it usually is.

Chapter Six

OXYCONTIN: PAIN FREE .... UNTIL YOU TRY TO QUIT

There is an addictive drug in America that is ripping through the social fabric of our country like a runaway locomotive. Whole communities of people are being torn apart, individual lives are being destroyed, and people are dying or committing suicide by the thousands. Those who don't end up dead may have to spend weeks or months in hospitals, and/or treatments centers trying to get off this monstrous drug. It grabs its users in a iron tight grip of addition, and won't let go. Cost for getting off the hook can reach tens of thousands of dollars. Some who do get free of the drug only relapse later and become more dependent than ever.

What is this horrible drug? It is heroin? Cocaine? Marijuana? Crack? How about good old alcohol? It's none of the above.

No this drug is new, and you don't get it from a street pusher. You get it from your family doctor. The drug is the extremely popular pain killer Oxycontin. This drug is a time-release version of the much older, much more well known drug, oxycodone, often bottled under the name Percodan or Percoset. It has long been known that oxycodone is an extremely addictive drug, but Oxycontin is a new, far more virulent form of the prescription drug.

That's because drug abusers -- and ordinary people -- can do much more with it than they can ordinary oxycodone. If oxycontin is simply swallowed, it will provide pain relief for about 12 hours. Small amounts of the drug are released slowly into the human body over this 12-hour period. But just some small changes in the way the drug is taken can turn this slow, careful pain reliever into a powerful high that people will do just about anything to get again and again. If oxycontin is simply chewed instead of swallowed, the high can be similar to heroin or cocaine. If it is crushed up and snorted through the nose, the rush is immediate and extreme. An even more potent way to get a mind-numbing effect is to break the pills down with water, insert it into a hypodermic needle and inject it directly into a vein, much like heroin is taken by serious addicts. Today, thousands of people are doing all of the above. The result is the latest "drug of choice" among people susceptible to addition.

What's interesting and especially troubling about oxycontin is that is is turning many ordinary people into serious drug addicts -- people who otherwise would never consider taking an illegal drug like cocaine or heroin in a million years. Yet, some how, some way thousands of people are choosing to use their doctor prescribed oxycontin as a recreational drug. Perhaps most of the time they abused oxycontin out of simple curiosity. But oxycontin is so powerful, many people are instantly addicted after their first "hit." no matter how they decide to take it. Some people take it just the normal, prescribed way, yet they too develop a sudden addiction. Sadly, some of the people who get addicted are innocently trying to deal with chronic pain -- from migraine headaches and back pain, to pain caused by diseases, like cancer or arthritis.

So bad is oxycontin addiction, and so easy is it to fall into, the maker of the drug, Purdue Pharma LP of Stamford, Conn., is currently being   sued by at least 13 people who say they have become addicted to the painkiller and others who want to hold the company responsible for a wave of overdoses and deaths among abusers.

Ira Branham, a lawyer and state legislator from Pikeville, Ky., who is suing on behalf of three people and the estate of a dead woman recently said to the Associated Press:

"This drug has been like a cancer attacking the very fabric of our little corner of the world," he said.

Branham said the responsibility should *"fall on the shoulders of the company that was the genesis of this problem."* He also makes the observation that many of his plaintiffs said they received OxyContin legitimately and became addicted by taking the prescribed dose, and as directed. They did not crush it and snort it, or inject it. Still, other lawsuits will attempt to hold the company responsible for illegal use of the drug..

Not only are individuals suing the drug company that makes oxycontin, but a number of states are bringing their own lawsuits. The state's attorney's general, including that of West Virginia, alleges Purdue Pharma violated state consumer law.

"They were telling doctors that OxyContin was far less addictive than other painkillers in this class of drugs," said Doug Davis, an assistant attorney general in West Virginia. "Now, we have a lot of people addicted to OxyContin in West Virginia. So was that a misleading statement? Yeah."

Of course, Purdue Pharma denies it is at fault. A spokesman for the company, James Heins said that victims and addicts are using the drug illegally or improperly. Some doctors support this contention. For example Dr. J. David Haddox, senior medical director of Purdue Pharma, said the chances of someone becoming addicted when taking OxyContin as directed are extremely small. He told the Associated Press:

"A lot of these people say, 'Well, I was taking the medicine like my doctor told me to,' and then they start taking more and more and more," Haddox said. "I don't see where that's my problem."

But Dr. Haddox's statement does nothing to explain away the many thousands of people who have become addicted to this hard drug. If oxycontin were safe and nonaddictive, why are thousands of people ruining their lives, committing suicide and faces years of super expensive rehabilitation if the drug is as safe and innocent as its makers claim?

Certainly, many people are abusing oxycontin and using it improperly. But many others are not. In either case, we see an example of a drug issued by a major, trusted drug company, which was also approved by the FDA. Whatever the cause of the major addiction problems developing across the United States, the fact remains that this drug is causing wide spread sickness, addiction and death.

Perhaps nothing is more valuable than information when it comes to oxycontin. Many people can still benefit from this drug, especially for those many people who suffer legitimately from chronic pain. Oxycontin is not a drug that will simply go away. The drug makes too much money for its makers. With this in mind, we are going to here provide a comprehensive guide to oxycontin and how you should use it -- or avoid it.

1. What kind of medicine is OxyContin?

As we said, oxycontin contains oxycodone, a very strong narcotic pain reliever similar to morphine. OxyContin is designed so that the oxycodone is slowly released over time, allowing it to be used twice daily. You should never break, chew, or crush the OxyContin tablet since this causes a large amount of oxycodone to be released from the tablet all at once, potentially resulting in a dangerous or fatal drug overdose.

2. What kind of pain is appropriate to treat with OxyContin?

OxyContin is intended to help relieve pain that is moderate to severe in intensity, when that pain is present all the time, and expected to continue for a long time. This level of pain severity may be caused by a variety of different medical conditions.

3. How do you know if I have the right kind of pain to use OxyContin?

Only a physician can determine if OxyContin is a good choice to manage a your pain. If you have pain every day that lasts for a large part of the day, and the pain is moderate or severe in intensity, depending upon other factors in your medical history, OxyContin may be a good choice for you. Speak with your physician. If you feel you only need to take a pain reliever occasionally and this adequately treats your pain, OxyContin is NOT the right drug for you. If you only need a pain reliever for a few days, for example following a dental or surgical procedure, OxyContin is not the right drug for you.

4. Are there any activities that you should not perform while using OxyContin for pain relief?

OxyContin may interfere with your ability to do certain things that require your full attention. You should not drive a car, operate heavy machinery, or do other possibly dangerous activities while taking OxyContin.

5. What should you do if you still have pain after I take the

OxyContin?

Because OxyContin is a very strong medication, you should not adjust the dose without first speaking with your physician.

6. Can you take other medicines while you are using OxyContin for pain relief?

Combining OxyContin with some other types of medication such as sleeping pills, tranquilizers, and other pain medications may be dangerous due to the risk of interactions of these medications that can result in injury or death. You should speak with your physician before taking any other medicines with OxyContin. You should also tell your physician about all prescription drugs, over-the-counter drugs, and dietary supplements/herbal remedies that you are taking before starting OxyContin.

7. Can you drink an alcoholic beverage while you using OxyContin for pain relief?

You should not drink any beverage that contains alcohol while you are taking OxyContin. This includes beer, wine, and all distilled liquors. OxyContin and alcoholic beverages may have dangerous interactions that can result in serious injury or death.

8. Can become addicted to OxyContin if you take it every day?

OxyContin is only intended for moderate to severe pain that is present on a daily basis and that requires a very strong pain reliever. Patients with this type of severe pain condition require daily pain treatment. Taking OxyContin daily can result in physical dependence, a condition in which the body shows signs of narcotic withdrawal if the OxyContin is stopped suddenly. This is not the same thing as addiction, which represents a situation in which people obtain and take narcotics because of a psychological need, and not just to treat a legitimate painful condition. Physical dependence can be treated by slowly under the advice of a physician by slowing decreasing the OxyContin dose when it is no longer needed for the treatment of pain. Concerns of addiction should not prevent patients with appropriate pain conditions from using OxyContin or other narcotics for pain relief.

9. What should you do when you no longer need the OxyContin for pain relief?

When you no longer need OxyContin, the dose should be gradually reduced so that you do not feel sick with withdrawal symptoms. You should ask your physician for a plan on how to gradually decrease the dose and when to stop the OxyContin.

10. What about the press reports about the misuse of OxyContin?

OxyContin is a safe and effective pain medication when properly prescribed and used as directed. OxyContin has also been used as a drug of abuse. You should protect your prescription and your medication from theft and never give OxyContin to anyone else. You should destroy any left over OxyContin tablets that you may have once your physician instructs you to stop taking the medication.

11. Can you take OxyContin if you are pregnant, planning to become pregnant, or planning to nurse my baby?

Your should speak to your physician about the effects of drugs like OxyContin on an unborn or newborn child.

12. Are there any other special precautions you should take with your OxyContin?

Because there is a large dose of medication in each OxyContin tablet, you must be very careful to keep OxyContin stored in a secure location, out of the reach of children. When you no longer need OxyContin for pain relief, you should flush the unused tablets down the toilet.

Conclusions

The sad story of oxycontin is just another among a long string of addictive drugs that have burst on the American scene, and have left lasting problems which take years to deal with, and often are never curbed entirely. For example, oxycontin's older cousin, oxycodone, sold as Percodan and Percoset, has been addicting people for decades on end. There has never been a successful way to stop getting this drug into the hands of those who are addicted and abusing it. The same could be said for dozens of other drugs, from Xanax and Tylenol with codeine, to Darvon and Ultram.

If you rely on "the system" meaning the FDA, doctors or other government agencies to protect you, you are relying on large complex bureaucracies that move slowly, get side tracked and even "bought off" by rich pharmaceutical manufacturers.

What this means is that you have to rely mostly on yourself. It is up to you to determine how you will take a drug, or whether to take it at all. It is also up to you to do your own thorough research on any drug you have been prescribed. This is far easier than you might think. You don't have to have any special knowledge of medicine or drugs. A simple search on any Internet search engine will provide you quick information on the drug you are considering using, including all the possible dangers and side effects.

Also, always consider an alternative, nondrug alternative, that is. In the example of oxycontin, which is a pain killer, there are certainly dozens of different ways to deal with pain -- from acupuncture and biofeedback -- to herbal remedies and milder, safer over the counter medications. Remember that when it comes to prescription drugs, knowledge is power. The more you know about the drug you are taking and its potential dangers, the better off you will be. You may even avoid death, addition or serious and permanent illness. A little research is well worth that final benefit.

Chapter Seven

NATURAL BORN KILLERS: Herbs that can sicken
or kill you

In the past 20 years or more there has been an explosion in interest in alternative medicine. So called "health food stores" have been popping up faster than mushrooms across the country and throughout the world. They offer a battery of herbs, vitamins, powered drink mixes, foods and dozens of other products -- all promising everything from a cure for cancer or depression, to more robust health for people who already enjoy normal health.

Perhaps the key word in "natural." Everyone believes that if it is "natural" it is automatically safe, healthy, and risk free. Nothing is more trusted than herbs, and herbal remedies. After all, herbs are just plants, many of them already extremely familiar to us. What could be safer than eating a lot of garlic every day to improve health? Or how about fish oil tablets? Certainly ordinary nutmeg is always safe to eat and risk free, right?

Well, the answer to all of the above is: "Not necessarily!"

Think about it. Poison Ivy Is Natural, Too! Just because a plant or herb is "natural" or unprocessed does not necessarily mean it's safe. Unlike prescription or over-the-counter medicines, herbs and other food supplements do not have to undergo review for safety or effectiveness before they are marketed. Some "natural" products, like herbs, may have powerful pharmacological effects that could present risks for people who take other medications or who have specific medical conditions.

It's not hard to be taken in by a promoter's promises, especially when successful treatments have been elusive. But the fact is that when it come to claims for health-related products, a healthy dose of skepticism may turn out to be the most promising prescription.

For example, did you know that ordinary nutmeg, when taken in doses of 5 grams or greater, can cause cause a person to have hallucinations, nightmares, blackouts, or periods of lost consciousness? It can. When you eat nutmeg normally, usually a teaspoon or less in a cake or other recipe, there is almost no chance of any harmful effect, unless you happen to be allergic to it. But nutmeg is also sold in most health food stores in pill or capsule form. Nutmeg when taken as a herbal remedy is said to heal or aid a variety of medical conditions.. But in a small percentage of people, the result can be bizarre hallucinations, frightening nightmares, even period of waking blackouts -- in other words, you can be up and around, walking and talking, without knowing it, or remembering any of it. Again, this reaction is rare -- but it is not so rare when many people decide to take mega-doses of nutmeg. They think: "Well, it's only nutmeg! My mother has been sprinkling it on cookies and baking with it for decades!" But the problem is that large, concentrated doses, especially when taken in pill or capsule form, bring a whole different, and possibly dangerous result.

What about garlic? Perhaps no other natural substance has enjoyed more popularity in the past 10 or 20 years than has this stinky root plant. If you listen to the radio at all, you have probably heard popular CNN talk show host Larry King boasting endlessly of the benefits of taking garlic. King, who suffered a major heart attack a few years ago, says he now takes garlic in pill form to lower his cholesterol and have a healthier heart. Garlic pills come in all shapes and sizes. Some people eat regular garlic daily on their foods, and then boost their intake by also taking garlic supplements in pill form.

Certainly, garlic offers many health benefits. It has been shown to be an effective cholesterol lowering remedy. It also is touted as a mild antibiotic, and an agent to keep the colon and stomach healthy and free of unwanted bacteria, especially yeast cells. Garlic is sometimes also suggested as a sleep aid. But can garlic be dangerous? Again, the answer is clearly yes, and again, the problem usually results from taking too much garlic, and when it is mixed with certain prescription drugs.

Sensitive people who eat too much garlic, or even a little garlic, may experience stomach cramps and other gastrointestinal disturbance. If you eat ten or more raw garlic cloves a day, you may poison yourself, or trigger an allergic reaction. Although yet to be fully verified, some experts say that garlic should not be used by nursing women because it can may cause colic-like problems in babies. The same anti-clotting properties that make garlic useful for lowering cholesterol and preventing heart attack prevention can pose difficulties for people at risk for stroke caused by blood vessel hemorrhage. Finally, garlic may be a significant blood thinner. That means if you take other drugs, such as aspirin, and other herbs, such as gingko, you are doubling up on blood thinning agents. This can lead to cuts that won't stop bleeding. Also, if you are scheduled to undergo any kind of surgery, including dental surgery, you could easily bleed to death if your doctor or dentist is unaware that you are taking blood thinning agents such as garlic and others.

A small amount of garlic taken daily will probably improve

your health, but taking large unnecessary amounts of garlic can cause everything from minor stomach cramps, to major problems with bleeding or worse. So use in moderation. Don't overdo it!

Now let's talk about another extremely common and very widely used natural substance -- aloe vera, the skin softening agent. Unless you have been hiding out in your basement for the past 20 years, you have certainly heard of the desert growing aloe vera plant, and it's naturally soothing sap that is highly valued as a skin softener and skin healing ointment, especially for burns and minor scrapes. Aloe can be found in dozens of different products these days -- in hand lotions, soaps, hair care products and more. Certainly something as gentle and healing and natural as aloe vera is completely safe, right? Wrong again. The fact is, aloe vera has been associated with a number of adverse reactions. First of all, you should never use aloe vera during pregnancy or while nursing a newborn infant. If you are having problems with intestinal obstruction, abdominal pain of unknown origin, or any inflammatory condition of the intestines, including appendicitis, Crohn's disease, colitis, irritable bowel syndrome, hemorrhoids, or kidney problems. Also, women should know that aloe vera should not be used for more than 8-10 days during menstruation. Finally, aloe vera is not recommended for children younger than 12 years old because it has been shown to cause fairly serious allergic reaction among the very young.

For years now, health experts have been touting the benefits of fish in the diet. Specifically, they have identified the fatty acid called omega-3, which is plentiful in many kinds of fish, especially salmon. Scientists have long observed that Eskimos and other people living in the frozen northlands have almost no incidence of heart disease. Their diet consists of large daily meals of fish and other seafoods. Thus, health experts have been recommending weekly, or even daily meals of fish for everyone to get the same benefits. But of course, the health food industry, smelling profits, rushed in to take the fish oil craze a step further. Today, consumers can find omega-3 fish oil sold in capsule form in health shops everywhere. Since most Americans do not care to eat fish every single day, they can still get their omega-3 by popping fish oil capsules. This is all well and good, but as it turns out, fish oil tablets have a significant blood-thinning property -- which is good for the heart -- but bad if a person is also taking other blood thinners, such as aspirin, and many prescription medications. People with arthritis, for example, take daily doses of a class of drugs called NSAIDS. These include drugs such as Naprosin, Indomethacin, Viotin and more. When NSAIDS are combined with fish-oil capsules, the results can be dangerous levels of blood thinning in the human body. This can result in bleeding problems, including stomach bleeding. Also, people can become faint and anemic, and thus be subject to fainting, light-headedness and weakness. If you are taking omega-3 fish oil capsules and you are also taking any kind of prescription medication, check with your doctor to be sure you are not doubling up on the effect these drugs are supposed to have on your body. In the long run, it's probably a much better idea to avoid fish oil tablets all together, and just eat a good meal of fish three to four times a weak. Remember, it's always much better to obtain healthy vitamins, minerals and fatty acids from their natural sources.

ST. JOHN'S WORT -- THE LATEST "MIRACLE HERB"

About two years ago, the popular ABC News program 20/20 did a major segment on a wonderful new herb that seemed to be more powerful than even the mighty Prozac in it's ability to treat depression. The herb was a very common folk remedy that had been known about and used in Europe for hundreds of year -- St. John's Wort. "Wort" is just another word for "flower." St, John's flower is a common plant which blooms with a yellow flower typically in the spring. When the flower is dried, crushed and processed into pill form, it taken as a food supplement or medication to treat the blues.

The 20/20 showed featured a number of people who had been depressed to the point of suicide, and who had received a number of more conventional treatments, only to remain deeply under the control of their dark moods. Even modern drugs such as Prozac and others had failed to produce significant results. Then the patients were put on a regimen of St. John's Wort, and according to the 20/s report, they were transformed. Their depression lifted, and they became just the opposite -- bright, happy, forward looking people who were finally free of gloomy, suicidal thoughts, and living productive lives.

The 20/20 report even told of a number of scientific studies conducted in Germany which strongly suggested that St. John's Wort was indeed a powerful anti-depressant. And so the case for St. John's Wort seemed to have been made. This natural herb that anyone could buy of the shelf, without a prescription, was the possible key to a happy, bright personality.

The day after the 20/20 report, sales of St. John's Wort exploded across the United States. Americans everywhere rushed to health food stores and bought every bottle off the shelf. Supplier of St. John's Wort could barely keep up with the demand. Because St. John's Wort was a "natural" substance, people assumed it was 100% safe, and they also began to swallow St. John's Wort capsules in large quantities. And for a year or two, everything seemed to be fine -- until problems started to crop up. Many people were mixing St. John's Wort on top of other prescription anti-depressant drugs they were already taking, causing all kinds of bad reactions. In some cases, the St. John's Wort counteracted the prescription drug, causing some people to become even more depressed, and even suicidal. Other people began to discover that St. John's Wort caused them to become hypersensitive to sunlight. Just a few minutes exposure to the sun could cause them to break out in a painful rash. Still other people developed serious mental problems and disorientation when they mixed St. John's Wort with alcohol, or even ordinary cheese. That's right! In some cases, mixing St.

John's Wort with cheese can produce negative side effects! Many other people discovered that St. John's Wort had no affect on them at all. After spending a few hundred dollars on the herb, they were left with thinner wallets, and more depressed than ever.

After a a couple of years, and millions of dollars in profits, studies began to trickle into the media spotlight that all the hype over St. John's Wort was just that -- hype. Yes, there had been a few small studies in Europe which suggested that St. John's Wort was an effective mood lifter, but more rigorous studies with larger numbers of people showed that St. John's Wort may have no more effect on depression than a glass of plain water -- if effect, no effect at all! Furthermore, St. John's Wort had some minor to serious side effects, resulting in sickness and more mental problems for a large number of people.

In fact, the National Institute for Health recently found some very deadly side between St. John's wort and an , a drug used to treat AIDS. NHI researchers recently demonstrated that St. John's wort could "significantly compromise" the effectiveness of HIV Protease Inhibitor.
The findings were detailed in the Feb. 12 issue of the prestigious British medical journal, The Lancet.

The report said: "When St. John's wort and the protease inhibitor indinavir are taken together, the levels of indinavir in the blood drop dramatically," said the study's principal investigator, clinical pharmacokineticist Dr. Stephen Piscitelli of the NIH Clinical Center's Pharmacy Department. "When the body eliminates the antiviral drug too quickly," he also said, there can be a loss of therapeutic benefit."

Another AIDS researcher, Dr. Judith Falloon of the Laboratory of Immunoregulation, National Institute of Allergy and Infectious Diseases (NIAID), added: "St. John's wort's effects on indinavir concentrations are large enough to be clinically significant. Patients and health-care professionals need to be aware of this interaction. Most people taking medications to treat HIV infection should avoid using St. John's wort."

The NIH Clinical Center study, conducted among eight healthy volunteers, first measured the amount in the body of the drug indinavir when taken alone. Next, study participants were given only St. John's wort for two weeks. Finally, indinavir and St. John's wort were given together.

"The results were dramatically conclusive," Piscitelli noted. "All the participants showed a marked drop in blood levels of indinavir after taking St. John's wort. The drop ranged from 49 percent to 99 percent."

"It's vital that we understand how drugs and herbal products interact," said Dr. John I. Gallin, Clinical Center director. "This research is important because it demonstrates that a common agent such as St. John's wort may have unsuspected adverse effects on the function of a drug essential to the health of a very vulnerable population."

Indinavir belongs to a class of drugs known as protease inhibitors. These drugs are among the most potent agents available for treating HIV infection and have been shown to prolong survival and slow the progression of the disease. Substances in both St. John's wort and in indinavir are thought to share a metabolic pathway, which suggested the probability of the drugs' interaction, Piscitelli said. The active ingredient in St. John's wort is suspected to induce drug metabolism, which revs up the rate the liver eliminates indinavir from the body.

The result is that there's not enough indinavir in the blood to do the job it's designed to do. "The low blood levels also can lead to drug resistance," said Piscitelli, who heads the Clinical Pharmacokinetics Research Laboratory at the NIH hospital.

"Resistance to indinavir can decrease the response to other protease inhibitors." They include nelfinavir, amprenavir, ritonavir, and saquinavir.

"Many people think that herbal products like St. John's wort are safe, but there can be dangerous interactions when taken with other medications prescribed to treat medical conditions," added Piscitelli.

"This study demonstrates how dangerous that interaction can be and how important it is for patients to keep their physician and pharmacist informed about any use of herbal products."

Adverse interactions also have been reported between St John's wort and cyclosporine, a drug used to reduce the risk of organ transplant rejection. Potentially dangerous changes in drug effects can occur when medications such as cyclosporine (Neoral, Sandimmune), digoxin (Lanoxin, Lanoxicaps) and warfarin (Coumadin) are taken with St. John's Wort extracts.

So, as you can clearly see, St. John's Wort is a "natural" substance that is far from harmless, and could be deadly in many situation. Overall, the jury is still out on St. John's Wort, and its supposed ability to treat depression.. Most likely, this herb has a small capability to lift the mood of people who are not seriously depressed,and in some cases, it may even be a good choice for people with true clinical depression. But the herb is certainly not the "miracle drug" that the media bandwagon made it out to be -- but by the time everyone sobered up and took a closer look at the products, millions in profits had been made and the damage was done both to the pocketbook of the consumer, and probably the healthy of many innocent people who put their faith in media excess and questionable drug company studies.

So here again we see an example of a relatively safe and common natural substance that somehow gets elevated into a kind of manic public craze which causes it to be used in an unsafe manner. With this in mind, let's talk about some general guidelines which consumers should use when it comes to using herbal supplements for health reasons.

When used in a common sense manner, herbal remedies are most often to be safer than conventional prescription drugs. They are more dilute, slower-acting and their side effects are usually less severe. Relatively few poisonings are reported each year because of herbs, and most of these are due to the consumption of toxic ornamental plants, not herbs. But clearly, herbal medicine is not risk-free, so some rules of thumb may help you use herbal remedies safely:

• Make sure of you match your health problem with the proper herbal remedy. An herb expert or "doctor" may be competent in the use of herbs to treat illness, but a
true medical doctor has the training and the tools to make an accurate diagnosis, and is also more competent at making sure you don't mix things up in a dangerous manner.

• Use according to label directions, unless directed by an herbal specialist. Don't over use! Once again, the temptation when dealing with "natural" herbal remedies is to believe they are completely safe, and that doubling up. or even taking 10 to 100 times the recommended dose is safe. Never make this assumption that a herb is not a "drug" even though it may not be, per se. But keep in mind, many of the modern pharmaceuticals you get from doctors are actually preparations based on natural planted-based products, many of them herbs. For example, the powerful heart medication, digitalis is derived from the common foxglove plant. If you are already taking digitalis, and you get a preparation from a herbalist that contains foxglove, you may be doubling or tripling the medication you are already on! That can result in serious sickness or quick death.

• Remember that herbs have their limits. Many natural food experts would have you believe that we would all be better off just dumping modern medicine and prescription drugs in the trash can, and go over to an all herbal health care system. If that ever happened, millions of people would die or be severely sickened. Yes, many prescription drugs are dangerous and deadly, but eliminating them in exchange for herbal remedies is not the answer. Herbs cannot treat everything, especially serious infections, acute medical conditions, and chronic diseases like diabetes. Insulin is the only known treatment for diabetes. While herbs may help improve a diabetic's overall condition, and perhaps even reduce the the amount of insulin needed, it will never replace it entirely.

• When it comes to herbs, knowledge is power. Before you take a single herbal supplement, learn all you can about it. Don't go to just once source, or trust one herbal expert. Cross reference your research with a variety of books, sources and medical opinions. That way you'll uncover any possible complications before you can do yourself any harm. If anything unexpected happens to you after you start using an herb, stop it right away. This includes even minor reactions, such as a rash or upset stomach. This could be a potential warning sign that this particular herb is not for you. Another common warning sign sometimes associated with herb is difficulty breathing. This is almost always a sign of an allergic reaction. The lungs swell and cannot take in enough oxygen. For a person with a heart condition or asthma, this could mean a quick death. Other common herbal reactions: headache, nausea, dizziness, light headedness, hot flashes, and more. If you experience any of the above, call 911 right away.

• Tell your doctor right away about any herb you decide to start using. Your doctor really needs to know. A recent report on ABC World News Tonight said that many people bleed to death during routine or even minor surgery because the doctor did not know that the patient was taking blood thinning herbs, such as garlic or gingko biloba. The herb you are taking may have no interactions with other drugs, but you can never be sure, so don't take that chance. Tell you doctor, even if you fear he or she will disapprove. You would rather face a little criticism from your doctor than end up losing your life over an accident that could easily be avoided.

• Don't just check out the herb -- check out the company which manufactures it and distributes it. Current law does not require that the FDA regulate the safety of herbal supplements. With no watchdog -- even an imperfect watchdog like the FDA --to monitor the safety of herbal remedies, you never know what you are getting. Just as we told you that the major drug companies are motivated by profits, so are many herbal producers. They are not immune to the huge cash potential that can be had from selling as many herbs as they can, whether they have been thoroughly tested for safety or not. Many independent studies have shown that the quality and safety of herbal products varies considerably from company to company. Also, consider this: many herbs come from underdeveloped counties in South America or elsewhere around the world. That means even herbs that are otherwise safe can contain impurities as they are packaged, including harmful bacteria, fungus and even other plants that get mixed into the vat. so to speak. One guideline is to look for the words "standardized extracts" on product labels. This will give you an idea about the strength and potency of what you are considering putting in your body.

• Some people seek to avoid the problem above by growing or harvesting their own herbs. But many people have eaten poisonous plants that they misidentified. Consider that some herbs may be edible only at certain times of the year. Also, one part of a plant may have medicinal value while another part may be toxic. What this means is that you must become an herbal expert yourself before you decide to grow and ingest herbs for medical purposes, or health benefits. Yes, you can trust yourself, but don't fool yourself. Get as educated as possible before you start growing, harvesting and using your own herbal products. Many herbalist spend years studying the long-range effects of herbs and all possible interactions and drawbacks. If you are not ready to make the commitment and do all the hard work, seek the advice and help of a trusted expert instead.

• A particularly potent way to take herbs is to buy preparations based on what is known as "essential oils." These are concentrations of specific volatile compounds found in plants. As such, they may be tens of hundreds of times more potent than the herb in its natural state. Many essential oil products can be used safely by skilled herbalists, but others can be very dangerous or even fatal when taken orally, even in cases where the raw plant material is considered safe.

With the above guidelines in mind, here are some more, specific contraindications for a few of the most popular herbal products. Contraindicated means that the substance should not be mixed with another herb, or with a specific prescription drug.

Be advised that herbal and other botanical ingredients of dietary supplements include processed or unprocessed plant parts (bark, leaves, flowers, fruits, and stems), as well as extracts and essential oils. They are available in a variety of forms, including water infusions (teas), powders, tablets, capsules, and elixirs, and may be marketed as single substances or in combination with other materials, such as vitamins, minerals, amino acids, and non-nutrient ingredients. Although data on the availability, consumer use, and health effects of herbals are very limited, some herbal ingredients have been associated with serious adverse health effects.

A. Chaparral (Larrea tridentata)

Chaparral, commonly called the creosote bush, is a desert shrub with a long history of use as a traditional medicine by Native Americans. Chaparral is marketed as a tea, as well as in tablet, capsule, and concentrated extract form, and has been promoted as a natural antioxidant "blood purifier," cancer cure, and acne treatment. At least six cases (five in the United States and one in Canada) of acute non-viral hepatitis (rapidly developing liver damage) have been associated with the consumption of chaparral as a dietary supplement. Additional cases have been reported and are under investigation. In the majority of the cases reported thus far, the injury to the liver resolves over time, after discontinuation of the product. In at least two patients, however, there is evidence that chaparral consumption caused irreversible liver damage. One patient suffered terminal liver failure requiring liver transplant.

Most of these cases are associated with the consumption of single ingredient chaparral capsules or tablets; however, a few of the more recent cases appear to be associated with consumption of multi-ingredient products (capsules, tablets or teas) that contain chaparral as one ingredient. Chemical analyses have identified no contaminants in the products associated with the cases of hepatitis. Products from at least four different distributors and from at least two different sources have been implicated thus far.

After FDA's health warning, many distributors of chaparral products voluntarily removed the products from the market in December of 1992. Some chaparral products remain on the market, however, and other distributors who removed their products from the market are seeking to clarify the status of these products.

B. Comfrey (Symphytum officinale (common comfrey), S. asperum (prickly comfrey), S. X uplandicum (Russian comfrey))

Preparations of comfrey, a fast-growing leafy plant, are widely sold in the United States as teas, tablets, capsules, tinctures, medicinal poultices, and lotions. Since 1985, at least seven cases of hepatic veno-occlusive disease--obstruction of blood flow from the liver with potential scarring (cirrhosis)--including one death, have been associated with the use of commercially available oral comfrey products.

Comfrey, like a number of other plants (e.g., Senecio species), contains pyrrolizidine alkaloids. The toxicity of pyrrolizidine alkaloids to humans is well-documented. Hepatic veno-occlusive disease following ingestion of pyrrolizidine alkaloid-containing products, has been documented repeatedly throughout the world. Hepatic veno-occlusive disease is usually acute and may result in fatal liver failure. In less severe cases, liver disease may progress to a subacute form. Even after apparent recovery, chronic liver disease, including cirrhosis, has been noted. Individuals who ingest small amounts of pyrrolizidine alkaloids for a prolonged period may also be at risk for development of hepatic cirrhosis. The diagnosis of pyrrolizidine alkaloid-induced hepatic veno-occlusive disease is complex, and the condition is probably underdiagnosed.

The degree of injury caused by pyrrolizidine alkaloid-containing plants, like comfrey, is probably influenced by such factors as the age of the user,body mass, gender, and hepatic function, as well the total cumulative dose ingested and the type of exposure (i.e., whether exposure was to leaves or roots, infusions or capsules). Infants in general appear to be particularly susceptible to adverse effects of exposure to pyrrolizidine alkaloids; there are reports of infants developing hepatic veno-occlusive disease following acute exposure of less than one week. Transplacental pyrrolizidine poisoning has been suggested by the occurrence of hepatic disease in the newborn infant of a woman who consumed herbal tea during pregnancy.

Although liver damage is the major documented form of injury to humans from pyrrolizidine alkaloid-containing herbals, animal studies suggest that their toxicity is much broader. Animals exposed to pyrrolizidine alkaloids have developed a wide range of pulmonary, kidney and gastro-intestinal pathologies. Pyrrolizidine alkaloid-containing plants, including comfrey, have also been shown to cause cancer in laboratory animals.

Four countries (the United Kingdom, Australia, Canada, and Germany) have recently restricted the availability of products containing comfrey, and other countries permit use of comfrey only under a physician's prescription.

C. Yohimbe (Pausinystalia yohimbe)

Yohimbe is a tree bark containing a variety of pharmacologically active chemicals. It is marketed in a number of products for body building and "enhanced male performance." Serious adverse effects, including renal failure, seizures and death, have been reported to FDA with products containing yohimbe and are currently under investigation.

The major identified alkaloid in yohimbe is yohimbine, a chemical that causes vasodilation, thereby lowering blood pressure. Yohimbine is also a prescription drug in the United States. Side effects are well recognized and may include central nervous system stimulation that causes anxiety attacks. At high doses, yohimbine is a monoamine oxidase (MAO) inhibitor. MAO inhibitors can cause serious adverse effects when taken concomitantly with tyramine-containing foods (e.g., liver, cheeses, red wine) or with over-the-counter (OTC) products containing phenylpropanolamine, such as nasal decongestants and diet aids. Individuals taking yohimbe should be warned to rigorously avoid these foods and OTC products because of the increased likelihood of adverse effects.

Yohimbe should also be avoided by individuals with hypotension (low blood pressure), diabetes, and heart, liver or kidney disease. Symptoms of overdosage include weakness and nervous stimulation followed by paralysis, fatigue, stomach disorders, and ultimately death.

D. Lobelia (Lobelia inflata)

Lobelia, also known as Indian tobacco, contains pyridine-derived alkaloids, primarily lobeline. These alkaloids have pharmacological actions similar to, although less potent than, nicotine. There have been several reported cases of adverse reactions associated with consumption of dietary supplements containing lobelia.

Depending on the dose, lobeline can cause either autonomic nervous system stimulation or depression. At low doses, it produces bronchial dilation and increased respiratory rate. Higher doses result in respiratory depression, as well as sweating, rapid heart rate, hypotension, and even coma and death. As little as 50 milligrams of dried herb or a single milliliter of lobelia tincture has caused these reactions.

Because of its similarity to nicotine, lobelia may be dangerous to susceptible populations, including children, pregnant women, and individuals with cardiac disease. Lobelia is nevertheless found in dietary supplement products that are marketed for use by children and infants, pregnant women, and smokers.

E. Germander (Teucrium genus)

Germander is the common name for a group of plants that are contained in medicinal teas, elixirs and capsules or tablets, either singly or in combination with other herbs, and marketed for the treatment of obesity and to facilitate weight loss.

Since 1986, at least 27 cases of liver disease (acute nonviral hepatitis), including one death, have been associated with the use of commercially available germander products in France. These cases show a clear temporal relationship between ingestion of germander and onset of hepatitis, as well as the resolution of symptoms when the use of germander was stopped. In 12 cases, re-administration of germander was followed by prompt recurrence of hepatitis. Recovery occurred gradually in most cases, approximately two of six months after withdrawal of germander. Analyses of these cases does not indicate a strong relationship between the dosage or duration of ingestion and the occurrence of hepatitis.

Although the constituent in germander responsible for its hepatic toxicity has not been identified, germander contains several chemicals, including polyphenols, tannins, diterpenoids, and flavonoids. On the basis of the 27 French hepatitis cases, the French Ministry of Health has forbidden the use of germander in drugs. Its use has been restricted in other countries.

F. Willow Bark (Salix species)

Willow bark has long been used for its analgesic (pain killing), antirheumatic, and antipyretic (fever-reducing) properties. Willow bark is widely promoted as an "aspirin-free" analgesic, including in dietary supplement products for children. Because it shares the same chemical properties and the same adverse effects as aspirin, this claim is highly misleading. The "aspirin-free" claim is particularly dangerous on products marketed, without warning labels, for use by children and other aspirin-sensitive individuals.

The pharmacologically active component in willow bark is "salicin," a compound that is converted to salicylic acid by the body after ingestion. Both willow bark and aspirin are salicylates, a class of compounds that work by virtue of their salicylic acid content. Aspirin (acetylsalicylic acid) is also converted to salicylic acid after ingestion.

All salicylates share substantially the same side effects. The major adverse effects include irritation of the gastric mucosa (a particular hazard to individuals with ulcer disease), adverse effects when used during pregnancy (including stillbirth, bleeding, prolonged gestation and labor, and low-birth-weight infants), stroke, and adverse effects in children with fever and dehydration. Children with influenza or chicken pox should avoid salicylates because their use, even in small doses, is associated with development of Reye syndrome, which is characterized by severe, sometimes fatal, liver injury. Salicylate intoxication (headache, dizziness, ringing in ears, difficulty hearing, dimness of vision, confusion, lassitude, drowsiness, sweating, hyperventilation, nausea, vomiting, and central nervous system disturbances in severe cases) may occur as the result of over-medication, or kidney or liver insufficiency. Hypersensitivity, manifested by itching, broncho-spasm and localized swelling (which may be life-threatening), can occur with very small doses of salicylates, and may occur even in those without a prior history of sensitivity to salicylates. Approximately 5 percent of the population is hypersensitive to salicylates.

G. Jin Bu Huan

Jin Bu Huan is a Chinese herbal product whose label claims that it is good for "insomnia due to pain," ulcer, "stomach neuralgia, pain in shrunken womb after childbirth, nervous insomnia, spasmodic cough, and etc." Jin Bu Huan has been recently reported to be responsible for the poisoning of at least three young children (ages 13 months to 2 2 years), who accidentally ingested this product. The children were hospitalized with rapid-onset, life-threatening bradycardia (very low heart rate), and central nervous system and respiratory depression. One child required intubation (assisted breathing). All three utlimately recovered following intensive medical care.

Although the product label identified the plant source for Jin Bu Huan as Polygala chinensis, this appears to be incorrect since preliminary analyses indicate the presence of tetrahydropalmatine (THP), a chemical not found in Polygala. THP is found, however, in high concentrations in plants of certain Stephania species. In animals, exposure to THP results in sedation, analgesia, and neuromuscular blockade (paralysis). The symptoms of the three children are consistent with these effects. An additional case of THP toxicity, reported in the Netherlands, appears to be associated with the same product, and is being investigated.

H. Herbal products containing Stephania and Magnolia species

A Chinese herbal preparation containing Stephania and Magnolia species that was sold as a weight-loss treatment in Belgium has been implicated recently as a cause of severe kidney injury in at least 48 women. These cases were only discovered by diligent investigations by physicians treating two young women who presented with similar cases of rapidly progressing kidney disease that required renal dialysis. Once it was determined that both these women had used the herbal diet treatment, further investigation of kidney dialysis centers in Belgium found a total of 48 individuals with kidney injury who had used the herbal product.

At the time that a report of these adverse effects was published in February 1993, 18 of the 48 women had terminal kidney failure that will require either kidney transplantation or life-long renal dialysis.

I. Ma huang

Ma huang is one of several names for herbal products containing members of the genus Ephedra. There are many common names for these evergreen plants, including squaw tea and Mormon tea. Serious adverse effects, including hypertension (elevated blood pressure), palpitation (rapid heart rate), neurophathy (nerve damage), myopathy (muscle injury), psychosis, stroke, and memory loss, have been reported to FDA with products containing Ma huang as ingredients and are currently under investigation.

The Ephedras have been shown to contain various chemical stimulants, including the alkaloids ephedrine, pseudoephedrine and norpseudoephedrine, as well as various tannins and related chemicals. The concentrations of these alkaloids depends upon the particular species of Ephedra used. Ephedrine and pseudoephedrine are amphetamine-like chemicals used in OTC and prescription drugs. Many of these stimulants have known serious side effects.

Ma huang is sold in products for weight control, as well as in products that boost energy levels. These products often contain other stimulants, such as caffeine, which may have synergistic effects and increase the potential for adverse effects.

II. Amino Acids

Amino acids are the individual constituent parts of proteins. Consumption of foods containing intact proteins ordinarily provides sufficient amounts of the nine amino acids needed for growth and development in children and for maintenance of health of adults. The safety of amino acids in this form is generally not a concern. When marketed as dietary supplements, amino acids are sold as single compounds, in combinations of two or more amino acids, as components of protein powders, as chelated single compounds, or in chelated mixtures. Amino acids are promoted for a variety of uses, including body-building. Some are promoted for claimed pharmacologic effects.

The Federation of American Societies for Experimental Biology (FASEB) recently conducted an exhaustive search of available data on amino acids and concluded that there was insufficient information to establish a safe intake level for any amino acids in dietary supplements, and that their safety should not be assumed. FASEB warned that consuming amino acids in dietary supplement form posed potential risks for several subgroups of the general population, including women of childbearing age (especially if pregnant or nursing), infants, children, adolescents, the elderly, individuals with inherited disorders of amino acid metabolism, and individuals with certain diseases.

At least two of the amino acids consumed in dietary supplements have also been associated with serious injuries in healthy adults.

A. L-tryptophan

L-tryptophan is associated with the most serious recent outbreak of illness and death known to be due to consumption of dietary supplements. In 1989, public health officials realized that an epidemic of eosinophilia-myalgia syndrome (EMS) was associated with the ingestion of L-tryptophan in a dietary supplement. EMS is a systemic connective tissue disease characterized by severe muscle pain, an increase in white blood cells, and certain skin and neuromuscular manifestations.

More than 1,500 cases of L-tryptophan-related EMS have been reported to the national Centers for Disease Control and Prevention. At least 38 patients are known to have died. The true incidence of L-tryptophan-related EMS is thought to be much higher. Some of the individuals suffering from L-tryptophan-related EMS have recovered, while other individuals' illnesses have persisted or worsened over time.

Although initial epidemiologic studies suggested that the illnesses might be due to impurities in an L-tryptophan product from a single Japanese manufacturer, this hypothesis has not been verified, and additional evidence suggests that L-tryptophan itself may cause or contribute to development of EMS. Cases of EMS and related disorders have been found to be associated with ingestion of L-tryptophan from other batches or sources of L-tryptophan. These illnesses have also been associated with the use of L-5-hydroxytryptophan, a compound that is closely related to L-tryptophan, but is not produced using the manufacturing process that created the impurities in the particular Japanese product.

B. Phenylalanine

A number of illnesses, including those similar to the eosinophilia myalgia syndrome (EMS) associated with L-tryptophan consumption, have been reported to FDA in individuals using dietary supplements containing phenylalanine. There are also published reports of scleroderma/scleroderma-like illnesses, which have symptoms similar to EMS, occurring in children with poorly controlled blood phenylalanine levels, as well as in those with phenylketonuria (PKU), a genetic disorder characterized by the inability to metabolize phenylalanine.

III. Vitamins and Minerals

Vitamin and mineral dietary supplements have a long history of use at levels consistent with the Recommended Dietary Allowances (RDA's) or at low multiples of the RDA's, and are generally considered safe at these levels for the general population. Intakes above the RDA, however, vary widely in their potential for adverse effects. Certain vitamins and minerals that are safe when consumed at low levels are toxic at higher doses. The difference between a safe low dose and a toxic higher dose is quite large for some vitamins and minerals and quite small for others.

A. Vitamin A

Vitamin A is found in several forms in dietary supplements. Preformed vitamin A (vitamin A acetate and vitamin A palmitate) has well-recognized toxicity when consumed at levels of 25,000 International Units (IU) per day, or higher. (Beta-carotene does not have the potential for adverse effects that the other forms of vitamin A do, because high intakes of beta-carotene are converted to vitamin A in the body at much lower levels). The RDA for vitamin A is 1,000 retinol equivalents (RE) for men, which is equivalent to 3,300 IU of preformed vitamin A, and 80 percent of these amounts for women.

The adverse effects associated with consumption of vitamin A at 25,000+ IU include severe liver injury (including cirrhosis), bone and cartilage pathologies, elevated intracranial pressure, and birth defects in infants whose mothers consumed vitamin A during pregnancy. Groups especially vulnerable to vitamin A toxicity are children, pregnant women, and those with liver disease caused by a variety of factors, including alcohol, viral hepatitis, and severe protein-energy malnutrition.

There are some studies that suggest vitamin A toxicity has occurred at levels of ingestion below 25,000 IU. In addition, the severity of the injuries that occur at 25,000 IU suggests that substantial, but less severe and less readily recognized, injuries probably occur at somewhat lower intakes. Most experts recommend that vitamin A intake not exceed 10,000 IU for most adults or 8,000 IU for pregnant and nursing women.

B. Vitamin B6

Neurologic toxicity, including ataxia (alteration in balance) and sensory neuropathy (changes in sensations due to nerve injury), is associated with intake of vitamin B6 (pyridoxine) supplements at levels above 100 milligrams per day. As little as 50 milligrams per day has caused resumption of symptoms in an individual previously injured by higher intakes. The RDA for vitamin B6 is 2 milligrams. Vitamin B6 is marketed in capsules containing dosages in the 100-, 200-, and 500-milligrams range.

C. Niacin (nicotinic acid and nicotinamide)

Niacin taken in high doses is known to cause a wide range of adverse effects. The RDA for niacin is 20 milligrams. Niacin is marketed in dietary supplements at potencies of 250 mg, 400 mg, and 500 mg, in both immediate and slow-release formulations. Daily doses of 500 mg from slow-release formulations, and 750 mg of immediate-release niacin, have been associated with severe adverse reactions, including gastrointestinal distress (burning pain, nausea, vomiting, bloating, cramping, and diarrhea) and mild to severe liver damage. Less common, but more serious (in some cases life-threatening), reactions include liver injury, myopathy (muscle disease), maculopathy of the eyes (injury to the eyes resulting in decreased vision), coagulopathy (increased bleeding problems), cytopenia (decreases in cell types in the blood), hypotensive myocardial ischemia (heart injury caused by too low blood pressure), and metabolic acidosis (increases in the acidity of the blood and urine).

Niacin (nicotinic acid) is approved as a prescription drug to lower cholesterol. Many of the observed adverse reactions have occurred when patients have switched to OTC formulations of niacin, and particularly when they have switched from immediate-release formulations to dietary supplements containing slow-release niacin formulations without the knowledge of their physicians.

D. Selenium

Selenium is a mineral found in dietary supplement products. At high doses (approximately 800 to 1,000 micrograms per day), selenium can cause tissue damage, especially in tissues or organs that concentrate the element. The toxicity of selenium depends upon the chemical form of selenium in the ingested supplement and upon the selenium levels in the foods consumed. Human injuries have occurred following ingestion of high doses over a few weeks.

IV. Other Products Marked as Dietary Supplements

A. Germanium

Germanium is a nonessential element. Recently, germanium has been marketed in the form of inorganic germanium salts and novel organogermanium compounds, as a "dietary supplement."
These products are promoted for their claimed immunomodulatory effects or as "health-promoting" elixirs. Germanium supplements, when used chronically, have caused nephrotoxicity (kidney injury) and death. Since 1982, there have

been 20 reported cases of acute renal failure, including two deaths, attributed to oral intakes of germanium elixirs. In surviving patients, kidney function has improved after discontinuation of germanium, but none of the patients have recovered normal kidney function.

One particular organogermanium compound, an azaspiran organogermanium, has been studied for its potential use as an anticancer drug. Forty percent of the patients in this study experienced transient neurotoxicity (nerve damage), and two patients developed pulmonary toxicity. Because of these side effects, medically supervised administration of this drug with monitoring for toxicity has been recommended for those using germanium chronically.

OTHER HERBS OF NOTE AND POSSIBLE PROBLEMS

• Black cohosh (Cimicifuga racemosa) -- Do not use during pregnancy or while nursing unless under the direct advice of an expert. Occasional gastrointestinal discomfort may occur, and large doses may cause vertigo, headache, nausea, impaired vision, vomiting and impaired circulation. Limit use to six months.

• Blessed thistle (Cnicus benedictus) -- Not to be used during pregnancy except under the direct advice of an expert. Large doses may irritate the stomach and cause vomiting.

• Cayenne (Capsicum annuum) -- Cayenne can be irritating to hemorrhoids. Do not apply cayenne to broken skin or near eyes. Prolonged application can cause skin irritation. If taken internally, do not exceed recommended dose -- high doses can cause gastroenteritis (inflammation of the gastro-intestinal tract) and kidney damage. While cayenne has been used as a treatment for ulcers, it can make matters worse under certain conditions.[6] If you have any digestive disorders, use cayenne only under the direction of qualified practitioner.

• Chaste tree (Vitex agnus-castus) -- Do not use during pregnancy except under the direct advice of an expert. Chaste tree may render birth control pills less effective. Occasional minor skin irritations have also been reported.

• Comfrey (Symphytum officinale) -- In the opinion of some experts, comfrey taken orally, has too many risks to justify its use. It may cause severe liver damage with long term use. If you do take it, don't do so for more than four to six weeks per year. Do not use during pregnancy or while nursing except under the direct advice of an expert.

• Feverfew (Tanacetum parthenium) -- Do not use during pregnancy unless by advice of expert. Mouth sores and stomach problems occur in a few users, usually in the first week of use. No long-term adverse effects are known.

• Ginkgo biloba -- This herb is generally very well tolerated. Ginkgo may potentiate MAO-inhibitors, so consult your physician if you are using an anti-depressant and are not sure if it is in this class of drugs. In large amounts, ginkgo can cause diarrhea, irritability and restlessness. Gingko is also well known to cause heartburn and stomach upset in many people.

• Goldenseal (Hydrastis canadensis) -- This should not be used during pregnancy. Do not take for more than two weeks at a time. Eating the fresh plant can cause inflammation of mucous membranes.

• Myrrh (Commiphora myrrha) -- Do not use when there is excessive uterine bleeding. Do not exceed recommended dose. High doses over a long period of time can be dangerous. If you are pregnant or have kidney disease, consult a physician before taking myrrh.

• Yarrow (Achillea millefolium) -- Do not use during pregnancy unless by advice of an expert. Some people may have allergic reactions to yarrow. With external use discontinue if skin irritation or itching occurs.

SPECIAL WARNINGS FOR THE ELDERLY

More than 60 million Americans who use herbal products, and the vast majority of them are elderly people. Furthermore, heath-care providers say that there has been a noticeable increase in this use among senior citizens in recent years.

But mixing herbs and prescription drugs is even more dangerous for seniors than for others because they tend to be in more frail health than younger people who can more easily fight off dangerous side-effects and recover from potentially bad reactions.

For example, drugs used to treat high-blood pressure, diabetes or heart disease -- all more common ailments as people get older -- should not be taken with products containing ginseng or ephedra (also called Ma Huang). Chemicals in these plants can increase blood pressure.

Also prevent strokes and other vascular problems, many elderly people take "blood-thinning" or anti-clotting drugs, including Coumadin (generic: Warfarin) and Plavix (Clopidogrel). The herbs feverfew and ginko biloba as well as Vitamin K should not be taken with "blood thinners."

"A lot of the elderly look for a quick fix," said pharmacist Ben LeCarre. "Seniors are more innocent. They are not accustomed to the mercinary and deceptive advertising that younger people take for granted these days. Seniors tend to simply believe what they've heard on TV or what they've read in an advertisement."

How to Spot False Claims

Just remember this: the first rule of thumb for evaluating any health claim is -- If it sounds too good to be true, it probably is! Also, be on the lookout for the typical phrases and marketing techniques fraudulent promoters use to deceive consumers. They include:

• The product is advertised as a quick and effective cure-all for a wide range of ailments.

• The promoters use words like scientific breakthrough, miraculous cure, exclusive product, secret ingredient or ancient remedy.

• The text is written in "medicalese"- impressive-sounding terminology to disguise a lack of good science.

• The promoter claims the government, the medical profession or research as a promotion for the product.

BEWARE OF ADVERTISING HYPE

If the advertisement for the product includes undocumented case histories claiming amazing results, you can almost bet that what they have is just another snake oil. Also beware if:

• The product is advertised as available from only one source, and payment is required in advance.
• The promoter promises a no-risk "money-back guarantee." Be aware that many fly-by-night operators are not around to respond to your request for a refund.

SPECIAL CLINICS IN FAR AWAY PLACES

Be wary of health care clinics that require patients to travel - and stay - far from home for treatment. While many clinics offer effective treatments, some prescribe untested, unapproved, ineffective, and possibly dangerous "cures." Moreover, physicians who work in such clinics may be unlicensed or lack appropriate credentials. Contact state or local health authorities where the clinic is located before you arrange an appointment.

WHY IT'S SO HARD TO RESIST

Health fraud is a business that sells false hope. It preys on people who are victims of diseases that have no medical cures, such as HIV/AIDS, Alzheimer's, arthritis, multiple sclerosis, diabetes, and certain forms of cancer. It also thrives on the wishful thinking of those who want short-cuts to weight loss or improvements to personal appearance. It makes enormous profits because it promises quick cures and easy solutions to better health or personal attractiveness.

The Most Common Some Medical Problems That Attract Health Fraud Schemes

• Cancer -- A diagnosis of cancer can bring feelings of fear and hopelessness. Many people may be tempted to turn to unproven remedies or clinics that promise a cure. Although some cancer patients have been helped by participating in legitimate clinical trials of experimental therapies, many others have wasted time and money on fraudulently marketed, ineffective and even dangerous treatments.

When you are evaluating cancer-cure claims, keep in mind that no single device, remedy or treatment is capable of treating all types of cancer. Cancer is a name given to a wide range of diseases that require different forms of treatment best determined by a medical doctor.

For more information about cancer you can trust, contact the American Cancer Society office listed in your yellow pages. To order free publications on cancer research and treatment, call the National Cancer Institute's Cancer Information Service at 1-800-422-6237.

• HIV and AIDS -- People diagnosed with HIV, the virus that causes AIDS, also may feel pressured to try untested "experimental" drugs or treatments. Although there are legitimate treatments that can extend life and improve the quality of life for AIDS patients, there is, so far, no cure for AIDS. Trying unproven products or treatments can be dangerous, and may delay proper medical care. It also can be expensive and usually, is not covered by insurance.

Don't be pressured into making an immediate decision about trying an untested product or treatment. Ask for time to get more information from a knowledgeable physician or health care professional. Legitimate health care providers will not object to your seeking additional information. The U.S. Government has established a toll-free HIV-AIDS Treatment Information Service, 1-800-HIV-0440. This information help line is staffed by health information specialists who are fluent in English and Spanish.

• Arthritis -- If you are among the estimated 37 million Americans who suffer from one of the many forms of arthritis, be aware that this disease invites a flood of fraudulent products and services. This is because medical science has not yet found a cure for arthritis. The Arthritis Foundation advises that symptoms should be monitored by a doctor because the condition can worsen if it is not properly treated.

Consumers spend an estimated two billion dollars a year on unproven arthritis remedies. Thousands of dietary and natural "cures" are sold for arthritis - mussel extract, vitamin pills, desiccated liver pills, shark cartilage, and honey and vinegar mixtures. Many supplements marketed as arthritis remedies are not backed by adequate science to determine whether or not they offer any relief. For a free brochure about unproven remedies, call the

Arthritis Foundation, toll-free, 1-800-283-7800 (9:00 a.m.-7:00 p.m., Eastern Time, Monday-Friday), or write: Arthritis Foundation, P.O. Box 19000, Atlanta, Georgia, 30326.

Precautions for Taking Dietary Supplements

Thousands of dietary supplements are on the market. Many contain vitamins and minerals to supplement the amounts of these nutrients that people get from the food they eat. There also are many products on the market that contain other substances like high-potency free amino acids, botanicals, enzymes, herbs, animal extracts, and bioflavanoids.

The FDA's review of the safety and efficacy of these products is significantly less than for drugs and other products it regulates. Be cautious about using any supplement that claims to treat, prevent or cure a serious disease. The FDA has approved only a few claims for labeling, based on a review of the scientific evidence (for example, claims about folic acid and a decreased risk of neural tube defect-affected pregnancies). The FDA allows other disease claims on supplement labels only if they are based on authoritative statements from scientific organizations such as the National Academy of Sciences.

Some dietary supplements have documented benefits; the advantages of others are unproven and claims about those products may be false or misleading. For example, claims that you can eat all you want and lose weight effortlessly are not true. To lose weight, you must lower your calorie intake or increase your calorie use through exercise. Most experts recommend doing both. Similarly, no body building product can "tone you up" effortlessly or build muscle mass without exercise. Claims to the contrary are false. Other questionable claims may involve products or treatments advertised as effective in shrinking tumors, curing insomnia, reversing hair loss, relieving stress, curing impotency, preventing memory loss, improving eyesight, and slowing the aging process.

In addition to lacking documented effectiveness, some dietary supplements may be harmful under some conditions. For example, many herbal products and other "natural" supplements have real and powerful pharmacological effects that could cause adverse reactions in some consumers, or cause dangerous interactions with other medicines. It doesn't necessarily follow that supplements marketed as "natural" are safe and without side effects. The FDA monitors reports of adverse reactions to dietary supplements to identify emerging safety issues.

According to the FDA, the following substances in dietary supplements are among those that can raise serious safety issues: chaparral, comfrey, lobelia, germander, willow bark, ephedra (ma huang), L-tryptophan, germanium, magnolia-stephania preparations and dieter's teas. In addition, some vitamins and minerals can cause problems for some people when taken in excessive doses. Finally, a label of "natural" is no guarantee of a product's safety or effectiveness.

If you use dietary supplements, always read product labels to determine the percentage daily value for various nutrients in the product. Also, it's a good idea to seek advice from a health professional before taking dietary supplements, particularly for children, adolescents, older people or those with chronic illnesses, and women who are pregnant or breast-feeding.

Conclusions

In general, herbal remedies are many times safer than just about any prescription drugs you can buy or get from your doctor. But never assume that anything that is "natural" or that is sold in a health food store is automatically without harm. There are many such products that can sicken, or even kill you. Also, many such products form deadly interactions with prescription drugs. Most doctors never ask patients if they are currently taking natural or herbal remedies. If you are, make sure you tell your doctor about everything you take. Also, most herbal products only become dangerous when they are not taken as directed, or taken in mega-doses. So many people feel that if one supplement a day is good, 10 or a 100 may be ten times or a 100 times better. This could be a deadly mistake! Use common sense! Get all the facts, read up on what you plan to use and always double check with your doctor. Your very life may depend on it!

Chapter Eight

The Latest Trend: Prescription Drug Abuse

Many people find it easy to get addicted to prescription drugs, especially pain killers. Other times, people take their prescription drugs in an inappropriate way, leading to death and illness.

According to the 1999 National Household Survey on Drug Abuse, in 1998, an estimated 1.6 million Americans used prescription pain relievers nonmedically for the first time. This represents a gigantic increase since the 1980s, when there were generally fewer than 500,000 first-time users per year. From 1990 to 1998, the number of new users of pain relievers increased by 181 percent; the number of individuals who initiated tranquilizer use increased by 132 percent; the number of new sedative users increased by 90 percent; and the number of people initiating stimulant use increased by 165 percent. In 1999, an estimated 4 million people - almost 2 percent of the population aged 12 and older - were currently (use in past month) using certain prescription drugs nonmedically: pain relievers (2.6 million users), sedatives and tranquilizers (1.3 million users), and stimulants (0.9 million users).

Although prescription drug abuse affects many Americans, many troubling trends can be seen among older adults, adolescents, and women. In addition, health care professionals - including physicians, nurses, pharmacists, dentists, anesthesiologists, and veterinarians - may be at increased risk of prescription drug abuse because of ease of access, as well as their ability to self-prescribe drugs. In spite of this increased risk, recent surveys and research in the early 1990s indicate that health care providers probably suffer from substance abuse, including alcohol and drugs, at a rate similar to rates in society as a whole, in the range of 8 to 12 percent.

Prescription Drug Abuse in Senior Citizens

Prescription drugs abuse may be the most common form of drug problems among the elderly. Part of the reason is that elderly persons use prescription medications about three times as frequently as the general population and have been found to have the poorest rates of compliance with directions for taking a medication. In addition, data from the Veterans Affairs Hospital System suggest that elderly patients may be prescribed inappropriately high doses of medications such as benzodiazepines and may be prescribed these medications for longer periods than are younger adults. In general, older people should be prescribed lower doses of medications, because the body's ability to metabolize many medications decreases with age.

An connection between age-related deaths and abuse of prescription medications almost certainly. For example, elderly persons who take benzodiazepines are at increased risk for falls that cause hip and thigh fractures, as well as for vehicle accidents.

Cognitive impairment also is associated with benzodiazepine use, although memory impairment may be reversible when the drug is discontinued. Finally, use of benzodiazepines for longer than 4 months is not recommended for elderly patients because of the possibility of physical dependence.

Data from the National Household Survey on Drug Abuse indicate that the most dramatic increase in new users of prescription drugs for nonmedical purposes occurs in 12- to 17-year-olds and 18- to 25-year-olds. In addition, 12- to 14-year-olds reported psychotherapeutics (for example, painkillers or stimulants) as one of two primary drugs used. The 1999 Monitoring the Future survey showed that for barbiturates, tranquilizers, and narcotics other than heroin, the general, long-term declines in use among young adults in the 1980s leveled off in the early 1990s, with modest increases again in the mid- to late 1990s. For example, the use of methylphenidate (Ritalin) among high school seniors increased from an annual prevalence (use of the drug within the preceding year) of 0.1 percent in 1992 to an annual prevalence of 2.8 percent in 1997 before reaching a plateau.

COLLEGE STUDENTS TOO

It also appears that college students' nonmedical use of pain relievers such as oxycodone with aspirin (Percodan) and hydrocodone (Vicodin) is on the rise. The 1999 Drug Abuse Warning Network, which collects data on drug-related episodes in hospital emergency departments, reported that mentions of hydrocodone as a cause for visiting an emergency room increased by 37 percent among all age groups from 1997 to 1999. Mentions of the benzodiazepine clonazepam (Klonopin) increased by 102 percent since 1992.

THE DIFFERENCE BETWEEN MEN AND WOMEN

Studies suggest that women are more likely than men to be

prescribed an a prescription drug that will later be abused. Narcotics and anti-anxiety drugs are the most commonly abused, and in some cases, a whopping 48 percent more likely. But overall, men and women have roughly similar rates of nonmedical use of prescription drugs. An exception is found among 12- to 17-year-olds: In this age group, young women are more likely than young men to use psychotherapeutic drugs nonmedically.

In addition, research has shown that women and men who use prescription opioids are equally likely to become addicted. However, among women and men who use either a sedative, anti-anxiety drug, or hypnotic, women are almost two times more likely to become addicted.

FOUR SIMPLE QUESTIONS

Here are four direct, simple questions you should ask yourself about your own presscription drug use.

(1) Have you ever felt the need to cut down on your use of prescription drugs?

(2) Have you ever felt annoyed by remarks made by friends or loved ones about your use of prescription drugs?

(3) Have you ever felt guilty about the way you use prescription drugs?

(4) Have you ever used prescription drugs to calm down or as a " little lifter"?

If you can answer yes to even one of these, you may already be addicted to a particular prescription drug. If you can't quit on your own, you may need professional help. Don't worry, you won't be alone. Every year, thousands of people get addicted to their prescription drugs -- even people who have never been addicted anything before in their lives. That includes people who have never touched a drop of alcohol, or taken a single puff on a cigarette.

But years of research have shown us that addiction to any drug, illicit or prescribed, is a brain disease that can, like other chronic diseases, be effectively treated. But no single type of treatment is appropriate for all individuals addicted to prescription drugs. Treatment must take into account the type of drug used and the needs of the individual. To be successful, treatment may need to incorporate several components, such as counseling in conjunction with a prescribed medication, and multiple courses of treatment may be needed for the patient to make a full recovery.

The two main categories of drug addiction treatment are behavioral and pharmacological. Behavioral treatments teach people how to function without drugs, how to handle cravings, how to avoid drugs and situations that could lead to drug use, how to prevent relapse, and how to handle relapse should it occur. When delivered effectively, behavioral treatments - such as individual counseling, group or family counseling, contingency management, and cognitive-behavioral therapies - also can help patients improve their personal relationships and ability to function at work and in the community.

Some addictions, such as opioid addiction, can also be treated with medications. These pharmacological treatments counter the effects of the drug on the brain and behavior. Medications also can be used to relieve the symptoms of withdrawal, to treat an overdose, or to help overcome drug cravings. Although a behavioral or pharmacological approach alone may be effective for treating drug addiction, research shows that a combination of both, when available, is most effective.

Treating addiction o prescription opioids

Several options are available for effectively treating addiction to prescription opioids. These options are drawn from experience and research regarding the treatment of heroin addiction. They include medications, such as methadone and LAAM (levo-alpha-acetyl-methadol), and behavioral counseling approaches.

A useful precursor to long-term treatment of opioid addiction is detoxification. Detoxification in itself is not a treatment for opioid addiction. Rather, its primary objective is to relieve withdrawal symptom while the patient adjusts to being drug free. To be effective, detoxification must precede long-term treatment that either requires complete abstinence or incorporates a medication, such as methadone, into the treatment plan.

Methadone is a synthetic opioid that blocks the effects of heroin and other opioids, eliminates withdrawal symptoms, and relieves drug craving. It has been used successfully for more than 30 years to treat people addicted to opioids. Other medications include LAAM, an alternative to methadone that blocks the effects of opioids for up to 72 hours, and naltrexone, an opioid blocker that is often employed for highly motivated individuals in treatment programs promoting complete abstinence. Buprenorphine, another effective medication, is awaiting Food and Drug Administration (FDA) approval for treatment of opioid addiction. Finally, naloxone, which counteracts the effects of opioids, is used to treat overdoses.

Help With Addiction to CNS depressants

IMPORTANT! -- Patients addicted to barbiturates and benzodiazepines should not attempt to stop taking them on their own, as withdrawal from these drugs can be problematic, and in the case of certain CNS depressants, potentially life-threatening. Although no extensive body of research regarding the treatment of barbiturate and benzodiazepine addiction exists, patients addicted to these medications should undergo medically supervised detoxification because the dose must be gradually tapered off. Inpatient or outpatient counseling can help the individual during this process. Cognitive-behavioral therapy also has been used successfully to help individuals adapt to the removal from benzodiazepines.

Often the abuse of barbiturates and benzodiazepines occurs in conjunction with the abuse of another substance or drug, such as alcohol or cocaine. In these cases of polydrug abuse, the treatment approach must address the multiple addictions.

How To Get Off The Hook of Prescription Stimulants

Treatment of addiction to prescription stimulants, such as Ritalin, is often based on behavioral therapies proven effective for treating cocaine or methamphetamine addiction. At this time, there are no proven medications for the treatment of stimulant addiction. However, antidepressants may help manage the symptoms of depression that can accompany the early days of abstinence from stimulants.

Depending on the patient's situation, the first steps in treating prescription stimulant addiction may be tapering off the drug's dose and attempting to treat withdrawal symptoms. The detoxification process could then be followed by one of many behavioral therapies. Contingency management, for example, uses a system that enables patients to earn vouchers for drug-free urine tests. The vouchers can be exchanged for items that promote healthy living.

Another behavioral approach is cognitive-behavioral intervention, which focuses on modifying the patient's thinking, expectations, and behaviors while at the same time increasing skills for coping with various life stressors. Recovery support groups may also be effective in conjunction with behavioral therapy.

THE MOST COMMONLY ABUSED PRESCRIPTION DRUGS

Although many prescription drugs can be abused or misused, there are three classes of prescription drugs that are most commonly abused:

• Opioids, which are most often prescribed to treat pain.

• CNS depressants, which are used to treat anxiety and sleep disorders.

• Stimulants, which are prescribed to treat the sleep disorder narcolepsy, attention-deficit hyperactivity disorder (ADHD), and obesity.

MORE ABOUT OPOIDS

Opioids are commonly prescribed because of their effective analgesic, or pain-relieving, properties. Medications that fall within this class - sometimes referred to as narcotics - include morphine, codeine, and related drugs. Morphine, for example, is often used before or after surgery to alleviate severe pain. Codeine, because it is less efficacious than morphine, is used for milder pain. Other examples of opioids that can be prescribed to alleviate pain include oxycodone (OxyContin), propoxyphene (Darvon), hydrocodone (Vicodin), and hydromorphone (Dilaudid), as well as meperidine (Demerol), which is used less often because of its side effects. In addition to their pain-relieving properties, some of these drugs - for example, codeine and diphenoxylate (Lomotil) - can be used to relieve coughs and diarrhea.

Opoids workb y attaching to specific proteins called opioid receptors, which are found in the brain, spinal cord, and gastrointestinal tract. When these drugs attach to certain opioid receptors, they can block the transmission of pain messages to the brain. In addition, opioids can produce drowsiness, cause constipation, and, depending upon the amount of drug taken, depress respiration. Opioid drugs also can cause euphoria by affecting the brain regions that mediate what we perceive as pleasure.

Chronic use of opioids can result in tolerance for the drugs, which means that users must take higher doses to achieve the same initial effects. Long-term use also can lead to physical dependence and addiction - the body adapts to the presence of the drug, and withdrawal symptoms occur if use is reduced or stopped. Symptoms of withdrawal include restlessness, muscle and bone pain, insomnia, diarrhea, vomiting, cold flashes with goose bumps ("cold turkey"), and involuntary leg movements. Finally, taking a large single dose of an opioid could cause severe respiratory depression that can lead to death. Many studies have shown, however, that properly managed medical use of opioid analgesic drugs is safe and rarely causes clinical addiction, defined as compulsive, often uncontrollable use of drugs. Taken exactly as prescribed, opioids can be used to manage pain effectively.

MIXING OPIODS WITH OTHER MEDICATIONS

Although opioids are generally safe to use with other drugs only under a physician's supervision. However, they should not be used with other substances that depress the central nervous system, such as alcohol, antihistamines, barbiturates, benzodiazepines, or general anesthetics, as such a combination increases the risk of life-threatening respiratory depression.

CNS DEPRESSANTS -- ANOTHEIR SOURCE OF ADDICTION

CNS depressants are substances that can slow normal brain function. Because of this property, some CNS depressants are useful in the treatment of anxiety and sleep disorders. Among the medications that are commonly prescribed for these purposes are the following:

* Barbiturates, such as mephobarbital (Mebaral) and pentobarbital sodium (Nembutal), which are used to treat anxiety, tension, and sleep disorders.

* Benzodiazepines, such as diazepam (Valium), chlordiazepoxide HCl (Librium), and alprazolam (Xanax), which can be prescribed to treat anxiety, acute stress reactions, and panic attacks; the more sedatingbenzodiazepines, such as triazolam (Halcion) and estazolam (ProSom) can be prescribed for short-term treatment of sleep disorders.

In higher doses, some CNS depressants can be used as general anesthetics.

There are MANY CNS depressants, BUT most act on the brain by affecting the neurotransmitter gamma-aminobutyric acid (GABA). Neurotransmitters are brain chemicals that facilitate communication between brain cells. GABA works by decreasing brain activity. Although the different classes of CNS depressants work in unique ways, ultimately it is through their ability to increase GABA activity that they produce a drowsy or calming effect that is beneficial to those suffering from anxiety or sleep disorders.

Despite their many beneficial effects, barbiturates and benzodiazepines have the potential for abuse and should be used only as prescribed. During the first few days of taking a prescribed CNS depressant, a person usually feels sleepy an uncoordinated, but as the body becomes accustomed to the effects of the drug, these feelings begin to disappear. If one uses these drugs long term, the body will develop tolerance for the drugs, and larger doses will be needed to achieve the same initial effects. In addition, continued use can lead to physical dependence and - when use is reduced or stopped - withdrawal. Because all CNS depressants work by slowing the brain's activity, when an individual stops taking them, the brain's activity can rebound and race out of control, possibly leading to seizures and other harmful consequences. Although withdrawal from benzodiazepines can be problematic, it is rarely life threatening, whereas withdrawal from prolonged use of other CNS depressants can have life-threatening complications. Therefore, someone who is thinking about discontinuing CNS depressant therapy or who is suffering withdrawal from a CNS depressant should speak with a physician or seek medical treatment.

CNS depressants should be used with other medications only under a physician's supervision. Typically, they should not be combined with any other medication or substance that causes CNS depression, including prescription pain medicines, some over-the-counter cold and allergy medications, or alcohol. Using CNS depressants with these other substances - particularly alcohol - can slow breathing, or slow both the heart and respiration, and possibly lead to death.

MORE ABOUT ADDICTION TO STIMULANTS -- "UPPERS"

As the name suggests, stimulants are a class of drugs that enhance brain activity - they cause an increase in alertness, attention, and energy that is accompanied by elevated blood pressure and increased heart rate and respiration. Stimulants were used historically to treat asthma and other respiratory problems, obesity, neurological disorders, and a variety of other ailments. But as their potential for abuse and addiction became apparent, the medical use of stimulants began to wane. Now, stimulants are prescribed for the treatment of only a few health conditions, including narcolepsy, attention-deficit hyperactivity disorder, and depression that has not responded to other treatments. Stimulants may be used as appetite suppressants for short-term treatment of obesity, and they also may be used for patients with asthma.

Stimulants, such as dextroamphetamine (Dexedrine) and methylphenidate (Ritalin), have chemical structures that are similar to a family of key brain neurotransmitters called monoamines, which include norepinephrine and dopamine. Stimulants increase the amount of these chemicals in the brain. This, in turn, increases blood pressure and heart rate, constricts blood vessels, increases blood glucose, and opens up the pathways of the respiratory system. In addition, the increase in dopamine is associated with a sense of euphoria that can accompany the use of these drugs.

The consequences of stimulant abuse can be dangerous. Although their use may not lead to physical dependence and risk of withdrawal, stimulants can be addictive in that individuals begin to use them compulsively. Taking high doses of some stimulants repeatedly over a short time can lead to feelings of hostility or paranoia. Additionally, taking high doses of a stimulant may result in dangerously high body temperatures and an irregular heartbeat. There is also the potential for cardiovascula failure or lethal seizures.

Stimulants should be used with other medications only when the patient is under a physician's supervision. For example, a stimulant may be prescribed to a patient taking an antidepressant. However, health care providers and patients should be mindful that antidepressants enhance the effects of a stimulant. Patients also should be aware that stimulants should not be mixed with over-the-counter cold medicines that contain decongestants, as this combination may cause blood pressure to become dangerously high or lead to irregular heart rhythms.

Conclusions

In the case of prescription drug abuse, you may think the patient is more to blame than the drug maker, or the doctor that handed the pills out, month after month. But the truth is, in this case, all three take some blame. As we said, even people who have never had a drink or a smoke of anything in their lives fall prey to prescription drug addiction. Many people get addicted after taking their very first pill. It can truly be that easy, and addiction is that fast and powerful. But this is something doctors should know -- yet millions of people are getting addicted. Why do doctors keep handing out pills? A good question, and one deserving a lot of discussion and more than a little investigation. The drug companies also bear a lot of responsibility. The fact is, they have little incentive to deal with addiction since the more pills people buy, the more money they make. If someone is addicted to a particular drug, the bottom line is that it means more sales for the drug companies. Thus, it would be foolhardy to count on them to step up and take strong action to change things. That leaves it with you -- once again -- it always come back to you. Like a broken record, we keep coming back to that theme in this book -- you are the one who is responsible for your own health and well being. Not even your doctor is going to take all the necessary steps to see that you stay out of trouble with drugs. The responsibility is ultimately yours. You have the power to avoid problems of all kinds with prescription drugs, including the tricky problem of addiction. Take that power and run with it!

Chapter Nine

A Guide to Safe Prescription Drug Use

In this book you have learned that using prescription drugs can often be like playing Russian roulette. Most of the time, the medicine your doctor gives you will do you more good than bad. Yet, there is always a percentage of times -- depending on the drug -- that you can be killed, sickened for life, or go through a painful illness as a result of what you took. In addition, there is another monster always lurking around the realm of prescription drug -- addiction. Many drugs help you at first, relieving pain or lifting depression, only to have you become enslaved to that drug for years, or forever. Kicking an addiction can take thousands of dollars in hospital care and counseling, not to mention tremendous psychological anguish.

The only 100% effective way to avoid the dangers of prescription drugs it to never take them. Unfortunately, even for the most healthy people, this is all but impossible. EVen a healthy person will run into a health related problem now - step on a nail, contract an infection, catch a bad flu or be poisoned by something contacted innocently in the environment.

Other people have no choice but to take prescription drugs. People with diabetes, cancer, heart disease all obviously need to take medicine to save their lives, or to have a somewhat normal lifestyle. For these people, the risks of prescription drugs almost certainly outweighs the dangers. That does not mean they do not face the same dangers anyone does when they take a prescription drug. But for people with life threatening or chronic condition, the realm of choice has been taken away from them.

So the challenge is, how do we use and benefit from the literally hundreds of prescription drugs on the market, while at the same time, avoiding the possible disastrous consqeunces that can result? This question also hold true for over-the-counter medication anyone can get without a prescription from a doctor.

There is a lot you can do to keep yourself safe. In this chapter, we're going to tell you what to do to avoid the many dangers and pitfalls of using prescription and nonprescription drugs.

IT BEGINS WITH YOU

Many times in this book we have decried the lax attitude of the majority of people when it comes to prescription drugs. We as a nation have become too reliant on doctors, drugs and the giant coporations who manufacture them, and advertise them with a vengence. It's an attitude of unquestioning faith. There is also the idea of the "magic pill." Too many people think they can do anything they want -- maintain poor diets, smoke, forego exercise, and ignore a healthy lifestyle -- and then expect a doctor will give them a magic pill to correct anything that goes wrong. A prime example of this are the extremely dangerous cholesterol medication we discussed at length -- the statins. Statins, including Baycol, Lipitor and Zocor. These drugs have proven to be extremely effective in lowering cholesterol, and thus helping people avoid heart attacks, high blood pressure, strokes and other diseases. Yet, these drugs have now been proven to kill. That's because in addition to melting cholesterol, the statins also tend to dissolve healthy muscle tissue, causing muscles cells to foul the kidneys and kill people.

This is especially sad since there are much better, completely safe nondrug ways to lower cholesterol. It's as easy as adopting a low fat diet and getting daily moderately rigorous exercise. But many people find giving up their juicy steak, or even taking a daily two mile walk too unappealing. It's so much easier to pop a pill and expect all the bad habits of a life tiem can be erased without effort, without pain, and without giving up anything.

The same scenario can also be said of anti-depression drugs. Rather than doing the tough soul searching work of finding out what is causing the depression in the first place -- getting to the root of the problem -- millions of people are opting for magic pills that will clear a way depression no matter what the cause. The popular nickname for Prozac, the best selling antipdepressant in history -- is "liquid sunshine." This calls forward the idea, for example, that rather than taking time for a peaceful walk in a beautiful park on a sunny day, popping a pill to alter the brain chemistry is so much easier. The person does not have to do anything to change the circumstances that caused the depression in the first place -- a hateful job, a poor relationship, dealing with the death of a loved one or any one of a dozen other possible situations.

So the first thing Americans need to come to understand is that there ain't no such thing as a free lunch. There almost always a price to pay when a person decides to take a prescription drugs. It may treat a medical problem, cure a disease or ease pain -- but the side effects can be worse than the original probelm. Everytime anyone takes a prescription drug, they should ask themselves: "Okay, what will be the consequences or downside of taking this drug, Is it worth it?"

TOO MUCH TRUST

When people go to a doctor or take a drug, they tend to relinquish all control of their own bodies to the doctor or the drugs. They assume that all doctors are better able to tell what is going on inside them than they are themselves. They go come to a clinic with the attitude: "Okay, here I am. Fix me!" If something goes wrong, they sue the doctor or the drug company as if they took no part in the entire transaction themselves. But that is precisely what is happening. When you go to a doctor, you must get involved with your own treatment. You need to ask questions and talk about options and alternatives. (Note: we'll discuss how to just that in the next chapter!)

Before you take a drug, you must spend some time in the library or on the Interent to find out how other people have faired on the same mode of treatment. You need to find out how the drug will possibly interact with food, alcohol, tobacco or over-the-counter drugs. If you simply pop a pill and "trust" that someone else is watching out for you, sooner or later you are going to run into trouble. All drugs come with dozens of paragraphs of fine print, warning of side effects and potentially dangerous interactions. If you don'ty take the time to read this fine print, you are laying yourself open to possible death, or lifelong illness. Yes, the fine print that comes with drugs seems almost impossible to read or understand, but wading through it may save your life. When you look at it in that light, an hour or two educating yourself about the potential pitfalls of of the drug you plan to take is a very small investment indeed.

A THREE-POINT PLAN FOR TAKING CHARGE OF YOUR OWN HEALTH

Now let's talk about specific ways you can keep yourself from safe dangerous drugs or dangerous drug interactions. We'll start with three major, broad points:

(1) HOW YOU INTERACT WITH YOUR DOCTOR

In the business of prescription drugs, doctors are the big gatekeepers. They are the go-between man or woman that stands between you and the makers of prescription drugs. Prescription drugs are regulated legally this way for a very good reason. It takes a person with a medical degree -- which means a minimum of 10 years or more of study -- just to administer them properly. So dangerous are prescription drugs, the legal and medical controls placed around them is a major facet of how are health care system is structured. It used to be the case that a medical doctor was the only entity allowed to get prescription drugs into the hands of the layman. But recently, a new kind of healthcare professional has been joined to this priviledge. These are the nurse practioners, also called the "physcician's assistant." A "PA" as they are called is usually a registered nurse who has had at least five years of on-the-job experience, and who goes back to medical school for two-three years to become a kind of hybrid between a doctor and a nurse. Unlike an ordinary R.N., a PA is trained both in diagnosing illness, and in prescribing drugs. But a PA is limited as to what drugs they can prescribe. They do not have access to the entire pantheon of drugs in the pharmaceutical armories of the world.

The doctor, and sometimes the PA, have the legal authorty to select drugs for you. The thing to remember is that no doctor is perfect, and no PA is error free when it comes to prescribing drugs. No matter how well trained, they are still human beings, subject to error. It's inevitable. You need to remember that you have a right to know the risks and the potential benefits of the drugs you may be prescribed. You also have a right to know about the alternatives. Just about all doctors and PAs assume they have total power over you. Too many doctors treat the patient like a machine that needs to be fixed or "fine tuned." You need to disabuse this notion in your doctor of PA by taking an active role in your treatment. We'll discuss this at greater length in just a few pages.

(2) YOUR PHARMACIST -- ANOTHER IMPORTANT RELATIONSHIP

We have just said that doctors are the supreme gatekeepers of prescription drugs. But after the gate is opened, a vital secondary gate presents itself. This is the pharmacist, another professional who knows a heck of a lot about drugs. In fact, drugs is a subject they have been immersed in during 4-5 years of university training, and what they deal with evrey day of their professional lives. Many experts believe that pharmacists actually know more about drugs than the doctors themselves, and this if often true. Thus, a pharmacist becomes an extremely important resource for you as you deal with prescription drugs. The great thing about a pharmacist is that they are easier to contact than a doctor, and their advice is almost always free. You don't need to make an appointment or pay for a clinic visit to find out what you need to know about a drug. All you need to do is pick up the phone and ask for your pharmacist. They tend to be extremely helpful, and even happy to talk about drugs. Despite being busy professionals, pharmacists generally tend to appreciate being asked.

The pharmacists is an excellent "walking cross reference" to the information provided by your doctor. When you double check things with a pharmacist, you are greatly improving your chances of avoiding problems with drugs. Utilize your pharmacist. He or she is a terrific resource, and they also have a vested interest in making sure you get the right drug. They need you as a customer and your business. That means they'll do everything they can to help you out. Granted, not all pharmacists are saints. Some are downright evil. Indeed, as this book was going to press, a sensational story broke about a pharmacist in xxxx who was diluting chemotherapy drugs for cancer patients. He did it, by his own admission, purely to make money. He watered down his medications and pcoketes the savings. The result is that many people may now die, or see their cancer come back and get worse. We provide this tragic true story not to frighten you, but to instill in you the idea that you must take as much responsibility for your own use of drugs as the doctors and the pharmacists. Never trust totally! Or to revive and old Reagan Administration line: "Trust but verify!"

(3) Most prescription drugs come with what is called a drug disclosure statement, or label. This is a small insert filled with print so fine you'll need a magnifying glass to read it. We'll discuss the

drug disclosure statement later, but we want to tell you about another valuable source of information about the drug you plan to take. You can find it in any library. It's a large book called the Physicians Desk Reference. It is updated yearly and lists every drug on the market, along with fairly easy to read information about drug effects, interactions, warnings and just about anything you need to know about the drug you plan to take. Better yet, the PDR, as it is called, is not published by the drug manufacturers, In other words, it is an objective, unbiased source of information not tied to the profit motives of the big drug makers. On the other hand, the PDR also tends to be highly technical and difficult to read for the layman. Also, the PDR is sometimes influenced by doctors and drug companies, who actually don't want this kind of information to be easy to read for the average person. There reasons are not necessarily negative. Doctors fear that oversimplified language in the PDR will leads to thousands of patients getting the wrong idea or misunderstandings about prescription drugs, and as a result, will develop a more confrontational relationship with medical providers. There is more than a little truth to this idea. Still, as a consumer, you deserbe to know everything there is to know about the drugs you are taking. Sources like the PDR can be a valuable ally in that effort.

THE NEXT STEP ... A PERSONAL MEDICAL DRUG INDEX

If you take just one prescription drug, this next step may not be necessary. But if you take one prescription drug, and a number of over-the-counter drugs, and even a few herbal or natural supplements, this should include you too. But for people who take more than one prescription drug, making a personal medical index may just save your life.

A personal medical index is a chart, or merely a list that records every drug you are now taking, and beside it or under it, all the basic facts about the drug, including effects, side effects, drug interactions, food interactions, and so on. Its probably best to organize your information in a series of columns. On the left side of the page, list the name of the drug. Then in each column moving to the right, list the next element of information. Every member of your family should have one if they also take prescriptio drugs, and nonprescription drugs, and also herbal and natural supplements. Also record any special instructions you learned about each drug from your doctor or pharmacist. Record not only the brand name of the drug, but also the generic or chemical name of the drug. For example, if you list "Prozac", put its chemical name "fluxotine right beside it. Keep in mind that the chemical names of drugs are always the same., but the brand name can vary widely, and almost always differs from country to country. Using brand names only is not reliable and can lead to confusion and mistakes. And it's confusion and mistakes that leads to terrible consequences when it comes to prescription drugs. Put down the dosage size as well. Such information will be listed on your pill bottle. If it's not, ask your doctor or phramacist.

In another column, right down exactly why you are taking the drug. For example, you may list Lipitor. This is a high cholesterol medicine. So put next to Lipitor: "To lower my cholesterol."

In still another column, put down how long your doctor wants you to stay on the drug. You may not have an exact time period or date. As in our example of Liptor, you may be on it until your cholecterol goes below a certain level. In this case, records that exact information. For example, you may write: "I need to take this drug until my cholesterol level goes below 125."

Keep your medical index up to date. Be obsessive about recording anythign and everything in it you feel necessary. Leave some room for some "general comments" to record how the drugs makes you feels, or to describe any possible side effects the drug may be producing in you.

One you have your medical record, bring it with you to the doctor every time you go. Your doctor will probably be fascinated and impressed. It will also help him or her do his job better. Of course, doctors keep their own, very careful records on your treatment program, but as we have said elsewhere in this book, doctors almost never know about drugs and substances you are taking or using outside their sphere of influence. The biggest example is herbal and vitimin supplements. As of today, most doctors are ignoring these potentially powerful substances which can have life threatening interactions with the drugs they are prescribing for you.

DANGEROUS DRUG INTERACTION

Now let's talk more about the all important subject of drug interactions. Perhaps more deaths and serious illness is caused by one druh interacting with another in a dangerous or deadly way. As we said, unwanted drug interactions may make your drug less effective, cause unexpected side effects, or increase the action of a particular drug. Drug interactions fall into three broad categories:

(1) Drug-drug interactions occur when two or more drugs react with each other. This drug-drug interaction may cause you to experience an unexpected side-effect. For example, mixing a drug you take to help you sleep (a sedative) and a drug you take for allergies (an antihistamine) can slow your reactions and make driving a car or operating machinery dangerous.

(2) Drug-food/beverage interactions result from drugs reacting with foods or beverages. For example, mixing alcohol with some drugs may cause you to feel tired or slow your reactions.

(3) Drug-condition interactions may occur when an existing medical condition makes certain drugs potentially harmful. For example, if you have high blood pressure you could experience an unwanted reaction if you take a nasal decongestant.

Drug Interactions and Over-the-Counter Medicines

Never forget that an over-the-counter (OTC) drug is a drug! Tylenol is a drug! Aspirin is a drug! Benadryl is a drug! Alka-Seltzer is a drug! Because they too can be dangerous, OTC drug labels contain information about ingredients, uses, warnings and directions that is important to read and understand. The label also includes important information about possible drug interactions. Further, drug labels may change as new information becomes known. That's why it's especially important to read the label every time you use a drug.

The "Active Ingredients" and "Purpose" sections list: the name and amount of each active ingredient the purpose of each active ingredient. The "Uses" section of the label: tells you what the drug is used for helps you find the best drug for your specific symptoms

The "Warnings" section of the label provides important drug interaction and precaution information such as: when to talk to a doctor or pharmacist before use the medical conditions that may make the drug less effective or not safe under what circumstances the drug should not be used when to stop taking the drug

The "Directions" section of the label tells you: the length of time and the amount of the product that you may safely use any special instructions on how to use the product.

The "Other Information" section of the label tells you: required information about certain ingredients, such as sodium content, for people with dietary restrictions or allergies

The "Inactive Ingredients" section of the label tells you: the name of each inactive ingredient (such as colorings, binders, etc.)

The "Questions?" or "Questions or Comments?" section of the label (if included): provides telephone numbers of a source to answer questions about the product

Learning More About Drug Interactions

Talk to your doctor or pharmacist about the drugs you take. When your doctor prescribes a new drug, discuss all OTC and prescription drugs, dietary supplements, vitamins, botanicals, minerals and herbals you take, as well as the foods you eat. Ask your pharmacist for the package insert for each prescription drug you take. The package insert provides more information about potential drug interactions.

Before taking a drug, ask your doctor or pharmacist the following questions: "Can I take it with other drugs? Should I avoid certain foods, beverages or other products? What are possible drug interaction signs I should know about? How will the drug work in my body? Is there more information available about the drug or my condition (on the Internet or in
health and medical literature)?

Know how to take drugs safely and responsibly. Remember, the drug label will tell you: what the drug is used for how to take the drug how to reduce the risk of drug interactions and unwanted side effects

If you still have questions after reading the drug product label, ask your doctor or pharmacist for more information. Remember that different OTC drugs may contain the same active ingredient. If you are taking more than one OTC drug, pay attention to the active ingredients used in the products to avoid taking too much of a particular ingredient. Under certain circumstances — such as if you are pregnant or breast-feeding — you should talk to your doctor before you take any medicine. Also, make sure you know what ingredients are contained in the medicines you take. Doing so will help you to avoid possible allergic reactions.

Common Examples of Drug Interaction Warnings

The following are examples of drug interaction warnings that you may see on certain OTC drug products. These examples do not include all of the warnings for the listed types of products and should not take the place of reading the actual product label.

Acid Reducers -- Drug interaction information: H2 Receptor Antagonists (drugs that prevent or relieve heartburn associated with acid indigestion and sour stomach)

For products containing cimetidine, ask a doctor or pharmacist before use if you are: taking theophylline (oral asthma drug), warfarin (blood thinning drug), or phenytoin (seizure drug)

Antacids -- (Drugs for relief of acid indigestion, heartburn, and/or sour stomach) Ask a doctor or pharmacist before use if you are: allergic to milk or milk products if the product contains more than 5 grams lactose in a maximum daily dose taking a prescription drug. Ask a doctor before use if you have: kidney disease

Antiemetics -- (Drugs for prevention or treatment of nausea, vomiting, or dizziness associated with motion sickness). Ask a doctor or pharmacist before use if you are: taking sedatives or tranquilizers. Ask a doctor before use if you have: a breathing problem, such as emphysema or chronic bronchitis glaucoma difficulty in urination due to an enlarged prostate gland. When using this product: avoid alcoholic beverages.

Antihistamines -- (Drugs that temporarily relieve runny nose or reduce sneezing, itching of the nose or throat, and itchy watery eyes due to hay fever or other upper respiratory problems). Ask a doctor or pharmacist before use if you are taking:z sedatives or tranquilizers a prescription drug for high blood pressure or depression. Ask a doctor before use if you have: glaucoma or difficulty in urination due to an enlarged prostate gland breathing problems, such as emphysema, chronic bronchitis, or asthma. When using this product: alcohol, sedatives, and tranquilizers may increase drowsiness. Avoid alcoholic beverages.

Antitussives Cough Medicine -- (Drugs that temporarily reduce cough due to minor throat and bronchial irritation as may occur with a cold). Ask a doctor or pharmacist before use if you are: taking sedatives or tranquilizers. Ask a doctor before use if you have: glaucoma or difficulty in urination due to an enlarged prostate gland.

Bronchodilators -- (Drugs for the temporary relief of shortness of breath, tightness of chest and wheezing due to bronchial asthma). Ask a doctor before use if you: have heart disease, high blood pressure, thyroid disease, diabetes, or difficulty in urination due to an enlarged prostate gland have ever been hospitalized for asthma or are taking a prescription drug for asthma.

Laxatives -- (Drugs for the temporary relief of constipation). Ask a doctor before use if you have: kidney disease and the laxative contains phosphates, potassium, or magnesium stomach pain, nausea, or vomiting.

Nasal Decongestants -- (Drugs for the temporary relief of nasal congestion due to a cold, hay fever, or other upper respiratory allergies). Ask a doctor before use if you: have heart disease, high blood pressure, thyroid disease, diabetes, or difficulty in urination due to an enlarged prostate gland.

Nicotine Replacement Products. -- (Drugs that reduce withdrawal symptoms associated with quitting smoking, including nicotine craving). Ask a doctor before use if you: have high blood pressure not controlled by medication have heart disease or have had a recent heart attack or irregular heartbeat, since nicotine can increase your heart rate. Ask a doctor or pharmacist before use if you are: taking a prescription drug for depression or asthma (your dose may need to be adjusted) using a prescription non-nicotine stop smoking drug. Do not use: if you continue to smoke, chew tobacco, use snuff, or use other nicotine-containing products

Nighttime Sleep Aids -- (Drugs for relief of occasional sleeplessness). Ask a doctor or pharmacist before use if you are: taking sedatives or tranquilizers. Ask a doctor before use if you have: a breathing problem such as emphysema or chronic bronchitis glaucoma difficulty in urination due to an enlarged prostate gland. When using this product: avoid alcoholic beverages.

Pain Relievers -- (Drugs for the temporary relief of minor body aches, pains, and headaches). Ask a doctor before taking if you: consume three or more alcohol-containing drinks per day. (The following ingredients are found in a wide variety of OTC pain relievers: acetaminophen, aspirin, ibuprofen, ketoprofen, magnesium salicylate, and naproxen. It is important to read the label of pain reliever products to learn about different drug interaction warnings for each ingredient.)

Stimulants -- (Drugs that help restore mental alertness or wakefulness during fatigue or drowsines). When using this product: limit the use of foods, beverages, and other drugs that have caffeine. Too much caffeine can cause nervousness, irritability, sleeplessness, and occasional rapid heart beat be aware that the recommended dose of this product contains about as much caffeine as a cup of coffee.

Topical Acne -- (Drugs for the treatment of acne). When using this product: increased dryness or irritation of the skin may occur immediately following use of this product or if you are using other topical acne drugs at the same time. If this occurs, only one drug should be used unless directed by your doctor.

Chapter 10

THE TWENTY QUESTIONS TO ASK YOUR DOCTOR OR PHARAMACIST

If you had a migrain headache, why would you seek out a gastroenterologist, a doctor who specializes in stomach disorders?

Hundreds of people do! Why? Because some headaches are severe enough to cause vomiting and abdomincal aches, and many people assume that their stomach is the problem and not their head!

You can't always assume a doctor is going to tell you different. If you go to a doctor and complain of vomiting and stomach cramps, he/she may treat you for that when, in reality, you need something for a headache!

The above is just one example of how obvious medical problems can be misinterpreted.

The fact is, one of the most difficult things for any doctor to do is find to what's wrong with you. Diagnostics, as it is called, is a science in itself, and many books have been written on that subject alone.

In order for a doctor to provide you with the correct treatment or to prescribe the right drug, he or she has to have some way of communicating with you in a way that is clear, meaningful, and which leaves little room for misunderstanding. It's just common sense — if you don't give accurate information to your doctor, how can he prescribe the proper treatment? Let's take a closer look at this important subject.

Twenty Questions About Drugs Your Should Ask Your Doctor

Talking to your doctor and getting actively involved in your own treatment is crucial. When you walk into a doctor's waiting room, you do not leave all responsibility for yourself outside the door. Just the opposite: when you are with your doctor, you would be much better off if you put on the hat of a tough investigative journalist, or maybe a mistrustful police officer. We do not mean that you should develop a hostile relationship with your doctor, or automatically call into doubt everything he says. However, you should ask a lot of probing and tough questions. To help you get started, here are the top 20 question you should ask your doctor about prescription drugs:

(1)   What is the name of the medication you have prescribed to me? Also, get both the Brand name, and its generic or chemical same. For example, the chemical same for prozac is fluxotine hydrocloride. When you set out to do a little research on the drug, you will need both names to help you find out what you need to know.

(2) What result can I expected from this drug?

Many times, the doctor will only tell you the "good" thing the doctor is supposed to do for you. For example, if a person with acne is prescribed the drug Accutane, the doctor will say: "It will clear up your acne." But what you need to ask about are side effects! What are the side effects of Accutane? And remember, a "side effect" is an effect! The term "side effect" lulls some people into believing that such effects are somehow something less than a direct, full-blown effect. Consider that the side effects of Accutane have been determined to include birth defects and dead-born babies! This is more than a "side effect." It's a major, life-changing effect! So whether you are taking a drug that is considered safe, or a drug for a condition as mild as acne, always ask your doctor what the drug will do -- and "what else" it might do!

(3) Are there any non-drug alternatives to taking this medicine?

Doctors are in the business to help sick people get better, but doctors are also under tremendous pressure and persuasion by drug companies to "move their products." Thus, most doctors will automatically opt to prescribe a pill before they suggest anything else. A prime example is that of high cholesterol drugs. A doctor can easily "order" a patient to go on a low-fat diet and get daily exercise before they prescribe one of the deadly statins, drugs that have been shown to lower cholesterol, but also kill many people. Many drugs have safer, more natural alternatives. Your doctor may or may not be aware of them, or even believe in them, but it still won't kill you to ask about them -- and it also may save your life!

(4) How long should I take the drug before I report that it's not working?

In some cases, this may be difficult, or impossible. For example, even people with dangerously high blood pressure may feel perfectly healthy, and a low-blood-pressure medication will make them feel no different. In this case, you need to go back to the clinic on a regular basis to have your blood pressure checked. In other cases, it's easy to monitor results. For example, if you have acne, chronic back pain or can't sleep, you should know fairly quickly whether the drug is working or not. Just make sure you find out the average length of time you can expect results.

(5) What is the exact dosage I should be taking?

Pills and capsules come in all sizes and shapes, but you should never judge a pill by its size or look. A pill or capsule may contain 5 mg or 25 mg, or even a 100 mg -- and all be the same size to the eye. The reason for this is that pharmacists prepare medications by "compounding" them to different strengths. The dosage amount will be listed on your pill bottle, but you should ask your doctor anyway how many to take and how often. Do exactly as the doctor and pharmacist directs. Make sure you know your proper dosage and count your pills carefully.

(6) What time or times of day or night should I take the drug?

This is more important than you think. For example, the drug prednisone will most often be prescribed to be taken in the morning. Some people might think: "Oh well, I forgot my prednisone this morning. I'll just take it now at 4 in the afternoon." But this may be a serious mistake. Prednisone is a hormone, and taking it at the right time is necessary to match where your own bodily hormone levels are at at the time. The human body has it's own rhythms, with certain hormones rising and falling according to the bioilogical clock. Many medications are designed to ineract with natural biological chemicals at certain times of the day. So follow exact timing instructions. Also, if you miss the appointed time to take your pill, don't double up on the pills the next time. In most cases, its best to skip the dose you missed, and take your prescribed dose the next time. This may vary somewhat, so ask your doctor for specific instruction. A diabetic, for example, may have serious problems if he or she skips a dose, and then fails to take another before the next appointed time of ingestions or injection.

(7) How does the medication work?

Many doctors grow impatient when you ask them this question, or they give a vague answer. This is somewhat understandable, since many medication have very complex processes, and describing how they work may take a degree in medicine to understand. Also, just how or why some drugs work is not well understood. For example, the drug Depakote is an anit-seizure medication, but is sometimes prescribed to prevent headaches. Though studies show that people have seen headaches decrease while on Depakote, the excact mechanism is not well understood. Even so, you should ask your doctor to explain in as simple terms as possible how the drug will work. A good doctor will be able to couch the explanations in terms that you can understand. If they don't, you may consider not taking the drug at all.

(8) How does alcohol affect this medicine?

Just about any drug you can get from a doctor will have some interaction with alcohol. Why? Well, don't forget -- alcohol is a drug! A very powerful drug. Yes, even a light beer is a drug, and even one light beer can cause a major reaction with just about any potential prescription drug. To be 100% safe, you should never drink any alcohol when you are taking any kind of prescription drug, period. But if you still plan to drink, be sure to find out what dangers you face by asking your doctor. Don't be embarrassed! Your doctor needs to know if you plan to drink, even a glass of wine or a beer now and then. Not asking could mean the end of your life!

(9) What interactions, if any, will this medicine have with other medicines, be they over-the-counter medications, or other prescription medications.

Especially if you are seeing more than one doctor, you need to find out what your latest prescription will do when you mix it with one or more that you are already taking. Most doctors will automatically get this information, but don't trust your doctor to do his own job. Many people, for example, will see a dermatologist for a skin minor skin problem, and then visit a general practioner for other medical purposes. They may think: "Well, the dermatologist only gave me a skin cream. That's won't have any affect on a pill I might take." This is simply wrong thinking. Skin medicine IS MEDICINE. It is usually absorbed into your bloodstream and can alter your total body chemistry as much as anything you swallow or get injected.

(10) What interaction, if any, will this drug have with herbal products, or other "natural" remedies.

We've talked about this in the "Herbal Killers" chapter and we advise you to go back an read it, or read it again. Many, many herbal and natural products actually have very strong actions on the body, and interactions with prescription drugs. For example, fish oil tablets containing omega-3 can be deadly to people with diabetes who are taking insulin. Omega three has been shown to increase blood glucose levels simply because it is high in calories. Fish oil also thins the blood, so people taking daily aspirin for a heart condition, or people taking NSAIDS for arthritis may thin their blood even more. That's because aspirin and NSAIDS are already blood thinners. The result can be anemia, fainting, or even worse, a coma. But this is just one example. There are dozens of herbal and natural products that interact with prescription drugs. Discuss this with your doctor!

(11) What effect will food have on this medication?

Did you know that some foods can cancel the effect of a drug you are prescribed? They can, and do! On the other hand, some foods can drammatically increase the effect a drug is supposed to have. We have already told you how fish oil makes blood even thinner for people who are taking prescription blood thinners. If you are taking a drug to help or cure a condition, a food you eat may be canceling it out. That's not as bad as a food doubling the potency of a drug, but either way, you need to know what you're doing, what you're eating and all the possible consequences. Make sure you ask your doctor about possible food interactions. It's important!

(12) Do you have any special instructions for taking this drug?

The word "special" can encompass a lot of scenarios. That's why it's such a good question to ask! It can, for example, take care of the previous three questions, or even all of them. Still, the word "special" also invokes vagueness, so be specific. Ask about all possible scenarios, and if you don't feel you're getting much information, start getting specific by going down the very list of questions we are giving you right here.

(13) How long should I continue on this medication?

Here's an interesting story: An eldely woman with arthritis was prescribed a number of medications for her condition. One afternoon while traveling far away from her home, she experienced a large flare of pain in her right shoulder blade. She went to an emergency room and was prescribed the powerful pain killer oxycontine to take care of the pain. But one year later, her husband asked her why she was taking oxycontin every day. As it turns out, the flare up that had caused the pain in her shoulder had long since subsided, as is often the case with arthritis. The fact is, she no longer needed the pain killer. She checked with her doctor, and sure enough, he told her that oxycontin was meant to be taken on a short term basis only. So for one year, the woman was taking a superfluous medication. The only trouble now was, she had become addicted to it. When she tried to quit oxycontin, her entire world fell apart. She became nervous and experienced great headaches. She also became depressed and filled with anxiety. It took months of expensive therapy thereafter to wean her slowly off the drug. She was lucky. If she would have asked a simple question from the start -- "How long should I take this drug?" she would never had to go through the horrid pain and agony of a major addiction, not to mention saving hundreds of dollars on a medication she did not need.

(14) Is my prescription renewable?

Ask if your prescription is renewable, and if not, why not? Sometimes doctors hand out a single months worth, or less, of a medication for one simple reason: To get it refilled, you have to come back for another office visit. Most doctors get paid by the visit, so each time you have to come back, it's money in everybody's pocket except yours. The money comes OUT of your pocket. Other times, however, the doctor will give you only one fill on your prescription to make sure you come back for a blood test, or other tests, to determine the affects the drug has had on your system. But once it has been determined that the drug your are taking is safe for you, request it be refillable a number of times, or, call the doctor's office and get a refill order by telephone. This way, you cannot be charged for another office visit. You still should go in for a regular blood test or check-up, however, to monitor how the drug is affecting your body. The more you do it, the safer you will be.

(15) Is it okay to save any of this medication for future use?

A great and important question to ask! Most often, a doctor will suggest you take all of your pills until they are used up. To often, people stop taking a medication after they start feeling better, only to find out later they are not entirely cured. This is especially true with infectious diseases, such as tuberculosis. In fact, whole new untreatable strains of TB are being created in some areas by people who stop taking their medications before they are cured. The result is that the TB germ is given a kind of vaccination against the drug. The result is a new and deadly strain of TB. This has been happening primarily with homeless people in major urban areas. The trouble is, you don't have to be homeless to contract the new, stronger form of TB. Anyone can get it. Other medications may lose their potency after a few months or a few years. So if you save it "for later" it may not work, and you could end up being very sick. Other drugs change their chemical nature after a period of time, especially if they are stored in high temperature areas, or under othe conditions that could aid in altering their chemical signatures. There are some medications which have a long shelf life, and can appropriately be used at a later time. But don't guess. Always ask your doctor or pharmacist about the how long to keep your medicine, or when to throw it away.

(16) What side effects should I report, and which can be ignored?

Just about every medicine has at least one, or several, side effects. Many side effects that seem frightening can be normal and nothing to worry about. But just the opposite situation can be the case. A minor effect may be a warning sign that you are in for big trouble! In either case, it's good and comforting to know what to expect in terms of side effects. When you know what to expect, you are not working in the dark, so to speak, when it comes to your medication program. Knowing what side effects you may encounter gives you the power and knowledge you may need to save your life, or to simply not worry about what may be happening to your body.

(17) Where should I keep my medications?

Some drugs will stay active only if they are kept refrigerated. This is often the case with antibitotics, such as penecillin, which is derived from a living culture of certain molds. Just like a food, they could "go bad" if not kept cool. Other drugs are rendered inactive if kept in a place that's too hot. In this case, you may take your pill thinking you are safe. The result could be catastrophic, depeding on what condition you are being treated for. WHERE you store your drugs can be just as important as how and when you take them, so make sure you get the facts on this.

(18) What do I do if I miss my scheduled dose of this medication?

Again, many people who miss a dose decide to double up on the next dose. This is almost never a good idea! The result could be an overdose and then sickness of even death. Most of the time you will be directed to simply skip the dose you missed, and take your next pill at its appointed time. Sometimes, though, missing a dose may result in adverse reactions, as with people suffering from diabetes. A diabetic who misses a scheduled dose of insulin may not live to take his or hre next. Knowing when to take your dose and what to do when natural human failure occurs can make all the difference in the world when it comes to prescription drugs.

(19) Can I get this drug in a less expensive form?

It's truly incredible the difference a name can make when it comes to both prescription drugs and nonprescription drugs. You've heard that old saying: "You're just paying for the name." This is probably more true in the realm of prescription drugs than anywhere else. A prime example can be found in over-the-counter medications. Tylenol, for example, is acetomenophen. Very often, this same pain medication is sold simply as "non-aspirin pain reliever." The only difference between the first and the second is price. The drug sold as Tylenol is very often twice or three times the price as the very same drug in generic form. Very often, the name brand and generic brand sit right next to each other on the drug store shelf. All a consumer has to do is look behind the box and in the fine print find: ACTIVE INGREDIANT. This will tell you exactly what you are buying. Acetomenophen is the very same substance whether it is being sold under the name "Tylenol" or as "Non-aspirin pain reliever." The same is true for many other medications. For example, did you know that the allergy medication Benedryl and the sleep aid Sominex is one and the same drug? Again, turning to the ACTIVE INGREDIENT heading, you will find that both Benedryl and Sominex are diphenhydromine, or DHI. One is packaged as an allergy reliever, while the other a sleep aid. But it's all just marketing. Furthermore, generic versions of DHI are available, most often at half or less of the price of the name brand. Well, the same is often true for prescription drugs. It is your doctor who most often decides which one you get -- the name brand or the generic. Again, the only difference will be price, and the difference can be truly staggering. Prozac is now available as fluxotine, for example. You will pay only one-half or one-third as much for the latter. Make sure you ask your doctor if the cheaper generic version is available and you'll save loads of cash. In case you are worried that the name brand will be of higher quality, you should know that both name brand and generic MUST BE chemically identical by federal law. SO there is no good reason to by name brand drugs over generic. The only true difference is money.

(20) Can you explain the "drug disclosure" statement for me?

The drug disclosure statement is the tons of fine print language that usually comes with a prescription drug. Very often it's printed in extremely small print on one sheet of paper that is folded over many times. But needing a magnifying glass merely to see the print clearly is the least of your problems. The bigger problem is interpreting what the disclosure statement is saying. Drug disclosure statements are not meant for the layman to read. They are loaded with arcane technical language so difficult to understand that even a doctor or a pharmacist can have trouble figuring out what it says. Your doctor or pharmcist, who are usually extremely busy people, may balk and squirm at this request, but it will force them to go into greater depth about all the indications and contraindications associated with the drug in question. Reading the drug disclosure statement by yourself will almost certainly prove an exercise in frustration and futility unless you have a degree in biochemistry or medical pharmacology. This means you need an interpreter. That means a doctor or pharmacist.

TALKING TO YOUR DOCTOR

Now let's have a brief discussion on how you should talk to your doctor. The doctor-patient should not be a "master-slave" relationship, as it too often is. You are a human being, and your doctor is not an unfailing god. They make mistakes, and so can you. You will fare much better if you take an active role in your doctor-patient relationship. Here are 10 guidelines or tips to help you do just that

Tip One: Nothing is too personal!

Sometimes, being totally open and honest, even when your life depends on it, can be an incredibly difficult thing to do. Many people, for example, will be hesitant to confide to their doctor that they may have a sexually transmitted disease, or that a member of their family is having problems with delusions or insanity.

Remember that a doctor "sees it all" almost everyday. If you tell your doctor you think you might have syphyliss or herpes, he or she won't bat an eye. It is not their job to judge you! It's their job to heal you. In order to do that, they need the truth from you.

Tip Two: Don't try to diagnose yourself

Many people go to a doctor after having given a lot of thought to what they think is wrong with them. Many have even reached a conclusion in their minds about what's wrong with them. But you should let the doctor make his own decision. He or she does it every day for a living, has spent 10 year in school learning how to do it and has a lot of experience with discovering medical problems. (Note: don't take this too far, however. Always reserve yor right to question your doctor, even doubt him/her. Sometimes being too passive in a doctor-patient relationship is one of the worst ways to get to the bottom of your medical probelm.)

Tip Three: Be prepared with a complete, accurate family history

Sometimes a doctor's examination, blood tests, X-rays and other diagnostic devices aren't enough to provide a complete picture of what might be wrong with you. Telling your doctor about your family history may be the best source, and provide the key to a proper diagnosis, especially if there is a condition in your family that is genetically generated and has a high probablity of being repeated.

Tip Four: Don't use medical terminology with your doctor

A frequent source of improper diagnosis happens when a patient uses medical terms in the wrong sense. Talk to your doctor in simple everyday terms. These days we are all inundated with medical information from the media — books, magazines, newspapers, radio, television — and much of the time this can be a great source of misuderstanding of medical terms on behalf of the public. Remember, many medical programs are primarily venues of entertainment, not serious medical care.

Tip Five: A simple idea: Point to where it hurts!

A person complaining of a pain in the chest or stomach may be suffering from any number of ailments. The chest or the stomach are not particularly large surface areas, there are literally an infinite number of spots on any human body where a medical problem can be pinpointed. As we saw in Rule One above, a stomach ache can be the result of a pain in the head. A pain in the chest may by on the right side just below the shoulder blade, or on the left side just below the rib cage — but you doctor won't know until you acyually point to just the right spot!

Tip Six: Keep in mind unusual activities or circumstances

Have you been recently engaged in some activity or been somewhere you don't normally go? Have you eaten a new kind of food, or tatsed something you've never tried before. This may be the key to a sudden, mysterious change in your health. Think hard. Where have you been or what have you done differently recently that may have made you ill. If you can think of something, even if it seems irrelevant, tell your doctor about it. This my provide the very clue that is needed to solve the puzzle of what's wrong with you.

Tip Seven: Don't let your child describe his/her own symptoms

For obvious reasons, a child may have many reasons to mislead a docotor. Children are easily frightended and confused by medical people and environments, and they may say anything a parent or doctor wants them to say. Even more that adults, children may use terms they don't understand, which can add to the confusion.

Tip Eight: Let your doctor talk to your spouse

The one person most people will share their most private and personal feelings with is their spouse. Often times a husband or wife can be more objective about you than you can be about yourself. If you are facing a daunting medical problem and have had little success after talking to many doctors, have your spouse to a doctor in private. It's amazing how often this can lead to a more honest and accurate assessment of what is going on with a person's health.

Tip Nine: Don't be a doctor doormat!

Traditionally the doctor-patient relationship has been one of "master and slave." It shouldn't be that way. A doctor is not an omnipotent God that knows all. In the not-so-recent past, doctors were never questioned or second-guessed by anyone, including nurses, technicians, and least of all, the patient. This approach can be counterproductive for both you and the doctor. Respect a doctor for what they are and what they know, but don't be totally passive to their every statement or suggestion. Take an active part in your own diagnosis and decisions about your treatment. If you doctor doesn't care for your input — fire him! After all it's your body and yor life. Ultimately, you are the one who is in control, and you bear the responsibility for your health.

Tip Ten: If your doctor recommends surgery ALWAYS get a second opinion!

At times the number of unnecessary surgies done in this country reached epidemic proportions. The economic incentive for a physician to operate on you is great. Surgeries make doctors a lot of money. Doctors are human beings and they are not immune to the lure of bigger profits. Whenever a doctor recommends surgery, you should take the time and trouble to go to a another doctor for a fresh perspective. Avoiding an unnecessary surgery could save your life and save you thousands of dollars! It's worth the time to get a second opinion.

CHAPTER 11

THE TOP 50 PRESCRIPTION DRUGS

Here you will find the Top 50 drugs prescribed in the United States today, based on number of prescriptions given. We will look at them one at a time, describe their purpose, talk briefly about their potential dangers, and suggest alternatives.

IMPORTANT NOTE: Never stop taking or alter your current usage of prescription drugs without consulting your doctor first. Also, the dangerous side-effects listed for each drug may not apply to all who use them. The side effects listed are the "potential" dangers of each drug, although each drug has been shown to cause the effects listed here in at least some people.

ANOTHER IMPORTANT POINT: The alternatives we talk about

here are not meant to be a substitute for your current prescription drug regimen. Again, see you doctor before you make any changes, or stop taking your current prescription drug. Alternatives to prescription drugs are not always the best answer to your health care needs. These suggestions are merely provided as possible alternatives to prescription drugs, but only as directed by your doctor.

THE TOP 50

No. 1 -- **Premarine** -- This is estrogen, the female hormone that occurs naturally in the human body. It is the most prescribed drug in America. Premarine is prescribed for women experiencing menopause, osteoporosis, ovarian failure, breast cancer, prostate cancer in men, bleeding of the uterus, vaginal irritation, birth control and Turner's Syndrome.

Potential Dangers: Has been associated with increased chances of getting cancer, especially endometrial cancer. Women who smoke while taking this drug greatly increase chance of cancer. Premarine can also cause vaginal bleeding, breast tenderness, pain in feet and legs, rapid weight gain, sudden severe headaches and more.

Possible substitutes -- If Premarine is taken, many doctors will combine it with progesterone, which has shown to reduce the risk of cancer. But a natural substance that provides natural estrogen is tofu -- made from soybeans. Tofu and other soybean-based foods can supply large amounts of natural estrogen if eaten every day, or almost every day.

No. 2 -- **Trimox** -- This very frequently used drug is a from of penicillin, used to treat infections. It can kill bacterial infections, but not viruses. Thus, man people who think penicillin is needed for colds or flus are usually mistaken.

Potential dangers -- Trimox and other penicillins cause allergic reactions in about 5% of the population. Reactions can be as serious as death, or minor illness. Most people think penicillin is very safe, but this is a mistake. Also, penicillin overuse can lead to loss of resistance to more deadly infections and bacteria, including flesh eating microorganisms. Only use penicillin as a last resort, as determined by a doctor.

Possible alternative -- Garlic is said to have antibiotic properties, but is not nearly as strong as penicillin. People with serious infections should not assume garlic is a good substitute, although it may help with minor infections. However, the best way to deal with infections is to prevent them from happening in the first place. That means a healthy diet, with daily adequate amounts of vitamins A, D, E, C, B complex, and the minerals calcium, chromium, copper, iron, magnesium, manganese, molybdenum, selenium, zinc and beta cerotine.

No. 3 -- **Synthroid** -- Used for cases of underactive thyroid and other thyroid problems. Perhaps one of the safest of all prescription drugs. Very few problems and few if any deaths are reported as a result of this drug.

Potential Dangers -- Side effects are rare, but can include heart palpitations, rapid heart beat, weight loss, tremors, headaches, nervousness and a few more. Most can be controlled by adjusting dosage.

Possible alternatives -- None

No 4. -- **Lanoxin** -- This is digitalis, a drug derived from the foxglove plant. It is used for heart problems. Improves ability of heart to pump blood and control heart rhythm.

Potential Dangers -- At first this drug seemed extremely safe and reliable. From 1982 to 1992, the FDA received only 82 reports a year of bad reactions. Considering millions of prescriptions had been issued, this is extremely safe. However, when researchers checked computerized hospital records from the federal Medicare program, a whopping 202,001 cases of adverse effects were found. Each of these cases were bad enough to require hospitalization. It would seem this drug has serious problems. Discuss thoroughly with your doctor before you decide to take this drug.

Possible alternatives -- There are no specific natural remedies to recommend, but prevention is probably the best alternative. Keeping a heart healthy means weight control, healthy low-fat diet, no smoking and avoiding other bad habits. Regular exercise will strengthen the heart. Do all of the above and you may be able to avoid Lanoxin and its serious side effects all together.

No. 5 -- **Hydrocodone** -- This is a powerful pain killer and a narcotic. It is used to treat mild to moderate and sometimes severe pain all kinds -- from headaches to cancer.

Potential dangers -- This is one of the most addictive drugs in the world. Many who use it quickly become dependent on it. Many people take this drug recreationally -- that is, for its high and the feeling of euphoria is gives to the user. Even people who believe they have a great deal of self control find themselves quickly hooked on this powerful drug. There is a major black market for hydrocodone for people want to take if for reasons other than pain.

Possible alternatives -- There are many safe alternatives for dealing with pain, including accupunture, massage, meditation. Depending on the type of pain hydrocodone is prescribed for, there are many alternative herbal remedies. For example, feverfew is indicated for headaches. If you have pain, seek to deal with it naturally before you consider this risk of getting addicted to this very tricky medication.

No 6 -- **Prozac** -- Extremely high profile and popular drug used for depression, obbsessive-compulsive disorder and other psychological problems. Closely related drugs are Zoloft and Paxil. Very expensive in nongeneric form.;

Potential Dangers -- See chapter dedicated to Prozac in this book. Prozac is extremely controversial. Has been linked to causing violent and suicidal behavior. Is known to cause sexual dysfunction and a "zombie-like" feeling of having no emotions. Has more than 242 known negative side effects.

Possible alternatives -- There are many non-drug ways to deal with depression, including talk therapy, group therapy, lifestyle changes, spiritual work on the self and more. Many natural substances may work as well, or better, including St. John's Wort.

But how about a common sense approach to fighting depression, rather than turning to a pill? Maybe it's best to just keep it simple. If you feel bad — that's it then — you just feel bad. Don't go out and pay a psychologist $50 per hour for six months to reach the same conclusion, or experiment with Prozac and its 252 side effects! Just acknowledge it without trying to draw any deep meaning from it. You know how you feel. You may not know why — but maybe it's not that important if you haven't pin-pointed the exact cause just yet.

Of course, there may be some very obvious reasons why you are depressed. Perhaps someone you love has died or is seriously ill. Maybe you have terrible financial difficulties. Maybe you are physically ill. Maybe your pet has died. Maybe you think the world is going to hell in a hand-basket. Whatever the reason, you should ask yourself very frankly if you are willing to get rid of your depression. What are you going to do about it right now? Obviously, you can't bring back someone who has died, but you can find a way to cope with it and bring yourself back from your depression. Obviously, you can't fix your financial difficulties over night, but you can take one small step today that will move you toward solving the problem.

Try the HALT formula

HALT stands for "hungry, angry, lonely, tired." If you are feeling bad, there is a strong chance that one of the above is causing it. Let's look at them one at a time:

(a) Hungry — Improper nutrition can cause depression in many ways. If you don't get enough to eat, whether it's from poverty or just the fact that you forget to eat when you should, the result can be depression. Eating the wrong kinds of food can also bring you down. If you live on junk food and sweets, you are flirting with depression. Your brain needs a well-balanced diet to keep you happy and healthy, so if you treat your body like a dumpground for Twinkies, depression may be a warning sign that you need to clean up your act. More specifically, studies have linked low levels of vitamin B-6 to depression and obsessive-compulsive disorders. Vitamin B-6 is needed for your body to make a brain chemical called serotonin. Serotonin may be a major factor in depression, so getting enough of it and vitamin B-6 may really help you out.

Don't eat ...

Sweets are one of the worst things you can give to your sullen nature. Soothing your feelings with a chocolate sundea or a box of chocolates can really bring you down. When you eat refined sugar, your body reacts by pumping insulin into your bloodstream, and insulin can be a major mood downer.

(b) Angry — Are you really ticked off at someone, at something about your life, or maybe even at yourself? Unresolved anger, which has been pushed down and forgotten may be festering inside you somewhere, sapping your energy and causing depression. The way to deal with anger is to confront it and discharge it. And the only way to do that is to cut loose — but you must find a safe way to do it! If you are really ticked off at your husband, don't bash him in the head with a baseball bat! Bash a watermellon instead and pretend it's your husband. Or try punching a pillow or performing some sort of strenuous exercise. The point is, you need to blow off steam in a way that does not hurt yourself or others. Screaming at the tops of your lungs when your are alone can really get a lot off your chest. Having a good cry (as long as it does not become self-pity) can help you get it all out. Whatever method you chose, after you discharge your anger, your emotional self will be relieved of a heavy burden and your will be free to climb the ladder of happiness.

(3) Lonely — Some psychologists say that loneliness is the number one cause of emotional probelms in our country. Today, millions of people are lonely. Why? Well, any thorough discussion of that would lead us into a lot of complex areas, like the break down of the nuclear family, and so on, but let's stay grounded in our simple common sense approach.

Depression and loneliness go hand-in-hand. Human beings are social animals by nature. Some people like to be alone, but most of us need the comfort and support of family, friends and even pets. In fact, recent studies by Swedish researchers suggest that loneliness not only leads to depression, but also may take years off your life. Studies of Swedish men showed that early death rates are significantly higher among men who live alone, and who reported that they had no one to share troubling times with.

If you are depressed right now, take a look at your life and see if you have someone or some people that you can turn to when you are feeling down. If your are estranged from your family, a spouse or your children, maybe it's time to take the first step to patch things up. If you don't have a family, go out and make a new friend. You could also join a club or take up a sport that will introduce yourself to new people. Whatever you decide to do, getting rid of loneliness may be the very thing you need to do to beat your depression.

(4) Tired — Are you getting enough sleep? Being tired and run down is closely linked to a depressed mental state. An old saying goes something like this: "There's nothing in the world that a hot bath and a good night's sleep can't cure." Well, a good night's sleep may not heal two broken legs, but it can blow away your depression.

In our high stress lives, many of us lose track of just how much we sleep. It's safe to say that anyone who is depressed, and who is getting less than eight hours sleep per night, may be experiencing depression brought on by sleep deprivation. Simply paying more attention to how many hours of shut-eye you get every day may make all the difference in the world. It will give your body chemistry the chance it needs to re-balance itself. It will clear your mind and give you a fresh perspective.

And be aware: every person is unique and has sleep requirements that are individual to that person. Did you know that Albert Einstein slept 10 hours a night? If he got anything less, he felt dizzy, disoriented and unable to think during the day. On the other hand, another genius, Thomas Edison, never slept more than three or four hours per night. When it comes to sleep, are you an Einstein or an Edison? Find out. Try adjusting the number of hours you sleep until you feel comfortable with it. If you need 10 hours — then that's what you should get. If you don't think it's macho, or if you think sleeping 10 hours per night is being lazy you're sadly mistaken. Getting the proper amount of sleep your body requires is good, healthy common sense. It's true you will have fewer waking hours, but you'll burn brighter during those hours, you'll get more done, you'll make fewer mistakes — and you'll be happier. If you're depressed, go through the HALT formula.

TV -- The "Natural" Depressor -- Ever heard that statement? "Garbage in, garbage out." Even if you are lonely, turning to your television for comfort and companionship can be the worst thing you can do. First of all, it will isolate you even more because you'll be less likely to go out an make new friends. You'll soon be more lonely and miserable than ever. Second, studies show that television not only slows down the mind, it also slows down your body chemistry. Watching too much television sets you up mentally and physically to be depressed. TV is full of violent images and also images of fantasies and riches that are unrealistic, and which can never be achieved by the average person. TV makes you feel like a loser because real life can never match up to the unreal world of the small screen. Quitting television can be as difficult as quitting smoking so try to wean yourself gradually, or just quit cold turkey, but make the effort.

You may be "SAD"

Many people find that they feel great in the summer, but miserable in the winter. The problem may be SAD, or Seasonal Affective Disorder. This is a condition which results from reduced levels of sunlight. SAD is associated with the pineal gland, which is sometimes called "The Third Eye" is esoteric circles. The pineal gland is located directly between your eyes on your forehead. When the amount of sunlight striking the pineal gland is reduced, it produces less of certain brain chemcials which help maintain your mood. Fixing SAD can be a simple as getting more sunlight. How do you do that during the dark days of winter? Well, just about any health care supply store, and some health food stores, stock lamps which produce the same kind of light radiation that the sun produces. Sitting in front of this light for an extra hour in the morning before the sun comes up, or after it goes down, can mimic the effect of a longer, summer day. Your pineal gland will began kicking out the brain chemicals you need to take you from SAD to GLAD.

Avoid naturally depressing food and othre subtances:

Many drugs and foods are depressants. The big one, of course, is alcohol. A lot of people say they are "feeling good" when they have a couple of drinks. But ultimately, alcohol teaches your body chemistry the lesson of depression. Avoid alcohol and you'll keep a major mood suppressor off your back.

As we mentioned earlier, sweets, especially chocolate have chemicals within them associated with depression. Also, drinking too much coffee can cause depression because it causes you to urinate more. When you urinate more, you deplete your body of depression-fighting substances, such as potassium and vitamin B-6. So kick the coffee, eat a banana and cheer up!

No. 7 -- **Vasotec** -- Used to treat high blood pressure and congestive heart failure. Also used to treat diabetic kidney disease and high blood pressure in children. In the group of drugs called ACE inhibitors.

Potential dangers -- Is known to cause serious kidney disease. Can cause swelling in the face, lips, hands and feet. Can also swell the tongue and hinder breathing. Is probably more dangerous for seniors.

Possible alternatives -- Garlic is known to lower blood pressure and protect against heart disease. Also, many forms of meditation, yoga and breathing exercises lower blood pressure. A low fat diet or vegetarian diet can help lower blood pressure. Reduce stressful situations in life and find ways to be happy.

No. 8 -- **Zantac** -- Used for frequent heart burn and stomach ulcers. Was once a prescription drug only, but now can be purchased without a prescription over-the-counter.

Potential dangers -- Should not be used by people with liver or kidney problems. Can cause the liver disease hepatitis Can also lead to intestinal worm infections because it reduces the acids that kills such parasites. Can cause dizziness and confusion. Should be avoided by women who are pregnant or breast feeding.

Possible alternatives -- Avoid the need for this drug by maintaining a healthy diet. Avoid greasy foods and other food that give heartburn. Stop smoking, which is a major source of heartburn. Baking soda and water is also an effective acid reducer in the stomach. Also, such over-the-counter medications as Rolaids and other are less dangerous.

No. 9 -- **Albuterol** -- Used for asthmas and bronchial conditions.

Potential dangers -- Should be used with extreme caution by people with history of angina pectoris (chest pains) heart disease, high blood pressure, stroke or seizure, diabetes, thyroid disease, prostate disease or glaucoma. Also, if used too often, can lead to worsening of asthma condition.

Possible alternatives -- (a) Onion extract on guinea pigs has shown that is can be a major anti-asthma agent. Studies on humans have also show that onion extract inhibited bronchial asthma. While you may not have a bottle of onion extract handy, try chewing on a slice of onion to treat your bronchial asthma attack.

(b) Vitamin C Studies have shown that about one quarter of asthma suffers can relieve their symptoms with 500 mg of vitamin C. This is not a quick solution, but it will shrink the air passageway sooner.

(c) Climatize your environment and avoid those foods that may trigger you. Many asthma attacks are associated with allergies. If that's the case, you are likely already aware of the places, conditions and foods that make asthma attacks likely.

(d) Check your reaction to aspirin and aspirin-like drugs. These can be a major source of asthma attacks. Indomethicin, which is a commonly used an anti inflammatory for arthritis and others conditions, is also a likely asthma culprit. If you react to them, avoid them and use aspirin substitutes.

(e) Monitor your lifestyle changes. Your asthma condition will change if there's a change in your lifestyle due to environmental factors. Or, you may develop an intolerance to a certain drug or a sensitivity to a new substance. If you are taking any medications, tell you doctor or pharmasist about any asthma attacks you think may be associated with the drug.

(f) Remember, emotional stress can trigger asthma attacks. If that the case, maybe it's time for a "time out" and to find a quiet place to sit or lie down for a minute.

(8) Get an air filter for your home or bedroom. Avoid all situations that can cause asthma attacks. If you live in a polluted city, move to a cleaner climate. Do more aerobic exercises to strengthen the lungs. Also, try vitamin B6 supplement. Recent studies show that B6 may be very effective in lessening chances of asthma attacks.

No 10 -- **Coumadin** -- This is a blood thinner used for preventing heart attack and strokes. Also known as Warfarin.

Potential dangers -- Coumadin is closely related to a substance used for rat poison. This drug can cause gangrene, fatal internal hemorrhaging, hideous birth defects and allergic reactions bad enough to kill. The maker of Coumadin warns doctors that: "Cigarette smoking increases the risk of serious cardiovascular side effects from oral-contraceptive use. This risk increases with age and with heavy smoking...and is quite marked in women over 35 years of age." Blood clots, strokes and heart attacks are potential complications. With Coumadin it is important to keep your vitamin K intake relatively constant. Too much of this nutrient, found primarily in green vegetables, can interfere with the anti-clotting action of the drug, and too little might lead to excessive bleeding.

Alternatives -- There are many natural blood thinners, including garlic, ginkgo biloba and fish oil, or omega-3. Aspirin is also a blood thinner and is less dangerous than Coumadin. All of the above may not be powerful enough for people at serious risk of stroke or heart attack, but alternatives should be discussed with doctor before resorting to coumadin. Also, a healthy lifestyle of low-fat foods and plenty of exercise will help the heart and lessen the chance of stroke.

No. 11 -- **Prilosec** -- Popular drug used for stomach ulcers and frequent heartburn. Heavily advertised by drug companies on TV and in print publications.

Potential dangers -- Can have serious allergic reactions. Also cause headaches, diarrhea, stomach pain, nausea. sore throat, fever, vomiting, dizziness, rash, constipation, muscle pain, tiredness, back pain and coughing.

Alternatives -- Avoid foods that trigger heart burn. Choose a healthy lifestyle with lots of exercise. Favor fruits and vegetables over meats and fatty, greasy foods. Never smoke or use chewing tobacco. Also try baking soda and safer over-the-counter meds, such as Rolaids before resorting to the more dangerous Prilosec.

No. 12 -- **Zoloft** -- A close relative of Prozac, it is also a serotonine reuptake inhibitor. used to treat depression and other mental illness problems. Even used to treat PMS in women. See chapter on Prozac and heading in this section on Prozac..

Potential dangers -- Has all of the same side effects associated with Prozac, including violent or suicidal behavior. Can "white-wash" a person of all emotions and ruin ability to have orgasm or enjoy sex.

Possible alternatives -- Nondrug therapy, such as talk therapy or accupuncture. Meditation, yoga or work on spiritual issues can also lead a person out of depression without resorting to drugs. Changes of lifestyle, elimination of problems, such as bad marriages or relationships. Get a dog, a cat or move to a beautiful part of the world. Smell the roses, walk in the grass barefoot. Quit your high stress job, find a new job you love. You get the picture!

No. 13 -- **Procardia XL** -- Prescribed for angina pectoris, chest pains, high blood pressure, migraine headache prevention, asthma, heart failure, Reynaud's disease, kidney stone attacks, gallbladder stones, and premature labor.

Potential dangers -- This is among a group of drugs known as calcium channel blockers. Procardia was approved by the FDA on the basis of only short term studies. In 1995, a study showed that this drug and other calcium channel blockers can increase the risk of cancer and heart attack. They also may produce internal bleeding.

Possible alternatives -- Cultivate a healthy lifestyle, eating low-fat, high fiber foods, and freeing your environment of those things which can trigger headaches or asthma attacks. Acupunture and meditation may be excellent alternatives.

No. 14 -- **Norvasc** -- Another calcium channel. In the same category of drugs as Procardia XL above. Used for mostly the same things. See the warnings and possible alternatives mentioned above.

N0. 15 -- **Claritin** -- Very popular allergy medicine prescribed by the millions. Is sold in some countries without a prescription, including Canada, where it can be bought over the counter. Considered a mild drug and safe, but not without problems.

Possible dangers -- Some people are allergic to this drug. People with liver disease should not take it. Most common side effects are dry mouth, headache, drowsiness, dizziness and fatigue. Should not be eaten on an empty stomach. Dizziness is probably the first sign of a potenitally severe side effect. If you get dizzy after taking this drug, contact a doctor immediately. Should not be taken by pregnant women. This drug passes into breast milk.

Possible alternatives -- Get an air filter for your home or bedroom. Avoid all situations that can cause allergic reactions. Find out what you are allergic to and avoid those specific triggers. If you live in a polluted city, move to a cleaner climate. Do more aerobic exercises to strengthen the lungs. Also, try vitamin B6 supplement. Recent studies show that B6 may be very effective in decreasing chances of allergic reactions. Build up your immune system with a healthy diet, exercise, a low-stress environment and positive attitude.

No. 16 -- **Zocor** -- Heavily advertised drug used for lowering blood cholesterol. Among a family of drugs called statins.

Potential dangers -- Statins have recently been identified with as many as 31 deaths in the United States, and at least nine deaths overseas. Statins have been determined to dissolve muscle tissue in the human body and leach those tissues into the blood stream. The muscle cells poison the kidneys, sometimes leading to death. The most deadly statin is a drug called Baycol. Zocor is probably much safer than Baycol, but this is not guaranteed. Zocor is very dangerous if mixed with alcohol. Also dangerous to people with liver disease.

Possible alternatives -- The best way to reduce cholesterol in just about all people is to cut down on fatty foods and start a good exercise program. Stay away from greasy meats and favor fruits and vegetables. Stop smoking. Avoid coffee and caffeine. Also, fish oil and garlic supplements are known cholesterol fighters. They are many times safer if not overused. It makes little sense to rely on a possibly very dangerous drug like Zocor when so many goods alternatives are available.

No. 17 -- **Biaxin** -- This is an antibiotic used to treat minor infections of upper and lower respiratory tract. It is also used to treat ulcers and skin infections.

Potential dangers -- This drug is relatively safe as far as known, but can have severe side effects. Most problematic is development of severe bleeding in the colon and bloody diarrhea. Has other less severe side effects, including nausea, vomiting upset stomach, changes in sense of taste, stomach cramps, stomach gas and headaches. People who are allergic to this drug could have more serious reactions.

Possible alternatives -- Maintain healthy lung tissue with good nutrition. Strengthening the body's immune system will prevent respiratory infections from happening in the first place. Never smoke and avoid second-hand smoke. Vitamin A and beta-carotene are essential for the normal development of lung tissue. Beta-carotene is particularly effective in preventing respiratory infections. Also helpful is vitamin E and the B vitamins. Vitamin C is widely believed to help respiratory infections clear up faster, and without resorting to antibiotics.

No. 18 -- **Cardizem** -- Prescribed for angina pectoris, chest pains, high blood pressure, prevention of second heart attack and Reynaud's disease. A calcium channel blocker.

Potential Dangers -- Another of the popular calcium channel blocker drugs. These drugs have been associated with increased risk for cancer. Also, this drug may have severe side effects if used in combination with anti-psychotic medications. This drug slows the heart rate. Can result in heart stoppage in some people. Can cause low blood pressure, and people with heart failure can die if they take this drug. Also should not be taken by people with liver disease.

Possible alternatives --The Hidden Salt/sodium factor. Sodium and salt is associated with high blood pressure. It's one thing to put the salt shaker away, and avoid the obvious salty foods, such as potato chips and salted peanuts. But there are many food in your diet which you probably thought were — without question — safe and healthy. What about, for example, a bowl of cereal with milk? A good choice for someone with high blood pressure? No! Especially if the cereal is Cherrios, which has a sodium content higher than many snack foods, including potato chips! Even the milk itself has a high level of natural sodium. In fact, milk and many kinds of cheese are extremely high in sodium and should be one of the first things restricted from a diet adjusted for hypertension.

Other cereals contain a similar level of sodium to Cherrios , so make sure you read the ingredient label carefully. Speaking of reading labels, those seeking to avoid excess salt in their diets should read all food labels. Remember that ingredients listed as Na, MSG sodium citrate and nitrates are all equally important to avoid. So do your homework! Check those labels and don't assume that foods are okay simply because they don't taste salty.

But a hypertension diet is not all about avoidance and bland food. Two substances in particular have been show to dramatically reduce high blood pressure: potassium and calcium. Increasing your intake of potassium and calcium may help you defeat your battle with hypertension. **Note:** Many antacid pills now contains calcium, but many also contain high amount of sodium. Read the label!

Meditation -- Not Medication! --As it does for so many other physical ailments, just a few minutes a day of quiet meditation has been shown — scientifically — to have an extremely beneficial effect on hypertension.

Exercise-- Of course, exercise is one of the most effective treatments for high blood pressure. It also helps in weight loss, improved circulation of the blood and oxygenates your entire system. But stay away from weight-lifting or isometric exercises. In general, a healthy lifestyle and low-fat diet improves blood pressure and function of the heart without drugs. Avoid smoking and second hand smoke. Reduce your stress level. Take a long vacation or quit your high-pressure job. Meditate or take up yoga. Play golf, go jogging daily. Also, garlic, fish oil and aspirin can help prevent second heart attack while lowing blood pressure. An exercise program approved by a doctor will go a long way toward eliminating the need to resort to a drug like this.

No. 19 -- **Zestril** -- This drug is prescribed for much the same condition as No. 18 on this list. It is an ACE inhibitor. To treat high blood pressure, prevent second heart attack and to treat congestive heart failure.

Potential dangers -- Allergic reactions in unknown number of people, possibly leading to death. Can also cause very low blood pressure. Can lower white blood cell count and make people more susceptible to infections.

Possible alternatives -- See blood pressure tips in previous entry. Remmeber that a healthy lifestyle and low-fat diet improves blood pressure and function of the heart without drugs. Avoid smoking and second hand smoke. Reduce your stress level. Take a long vacation or quit your high-pressure job. Meditate or take up yoga. Play golf, go jogging daily. Also, garlic, fish oil and aspirin can help prevent second heart attack while lowing blood pressure. An exercise program approved by a doctor will go a long way toward eliminating the need to use this drug.

No. 20 -- **Augmentin** -- A penicillin antibiotic. Used to treat a wide variety of infections.

Potential dangers -- Biggest danger is allergic reaction, which can be minor, or a serious as death. This drug can counter the effects of oral contraceptives. If you don't want to get pregnant, don't take this drug while you are on the pill. Allergic reactions are made stronger by beta-blockers. May increase the effect of blood thinners, such as aspirin. If you take the drug with fruit juice or a carbonated beverage, it will not be effective. Not recommended for women best feeding, although the risk is small.

Possible alternatives -- Best way to deal with infections is to avoid them in the first place. That means developing a healthy immune system with a healthy diet, regular exercise and vitamin rich diet that includes high amounts of fruits and vegetables. Garlic in known to have antibiotic properties. Taking garlic on a daily basis may keep you from serious infection, but is not guaranteed.

No. 21 -- **Paxil** -- Another Prozac-like drug. Used for depression, diabetic nerve disease, headache and premature ejaculation.

Potential Dangers -- See chapter dedicated to Prozac in this book. Also see listing for Zoloft. Like Prozac and Zoloft, Paxil is extremely controversial. Has been linked to causing violent and suicidal behavior. Is known to cause sexual dysfunction and a "zombie-like" feeling of having no emotions. Has more than 242 known negative side effects.

Possible alternatives -- There are many non-drug ways to deal with depression, including talk therapy, group therapy, lifestyle changes, spiritual work on the self and more. Many natural substances may work as well, or better, including St. John's Wort.

No 22 -- **Amoxil** -- Another penicillin antibiotic.

Biggest danger is allergic reaction, which can be minor, or a serious as death. This drug can counter the effects of oral contraceptives. If you don't want to get pregnant, don't take this drug while you are on the pill. Allergic reactions are made stronger by beta-blockers. May increase the effect of blood thinners, such as aspirin. If you take the drug with fruit juice or a carbonated beverage, it will not be effective. Not recommended for women best feeding, although the risk is small.

Possible alternatives -- Best way to deal with infections is to avoid them in the first place. That means developing a healthy immune system with a healthy diet, regular exercise and vitamin rich diet that includes high amounts of fruits and vegetables. Garlic in known to have antibiotic properties. Taking garlic on a daily basis may keep you from serious infection, but is not guaranteed.

No. 23 -- **Furosemide** -- This drug is a diuretic which helps rid the body of excess fluid. It is prescribed for people with congestive heart failure, cirrhosis of the liver, fluid in the lungs, kidney problems, high blood pressure and more. This drug is called a "loop" diuretic because it affects a portion of the kidney called the "loop of Henle."

Potential Dangers -- Can cause minor to severe allergic reactions. Can cause severe dehydration and lower electrolyte levels in the body. Can also reduce the volume of blood in the body. They can also cause some people to loose their hearing. Some people experience ringing in the ears, a feeling of fullness in the ears and fainting. This drug may increase cholesterol levels in some people. Because it reduces electrolytes, people may become weak and dizzy, have dry mouth, be subject to passing out and may become more susceptible to other diseases and infections.

Possible alternatives -- There are many natural diuretics, including any drink that contains caffeine, such as coffee and soft drinks. These may not be appropriate substitutes, however, for people with major fluid retention problems. You will probably not be using this drug unless you have a great need for it, such as heart disease or major fluid build-up in the lungs due to lung cancer or other lung diseases. Discuss other possible alternatives with your doctor. Some diuretic are safer than others.

No. 24 -- **Triamterene** -- Another diuretic drug. Used to help eliminate excess fluids from the body. It may be safer than Furosemide because it does not deplete the body of potassium as does Furosemide.

Potential dangers -- Do not take with a potassium supplement or adverse reactions may occur. Can cause allergic reactions. Can cause dizziness, appetite loss, drowsiness, stomach upset and diarrhea.

Possible alternatives -- There are many natural diuretics, including any drink that contains caffeine, such as coffee and soft drinks. These may not be appropriate substitutes, however, for people with major fluid retention problems. You will probably not be using this drug unless you have a great need for it, such as heart disease or major fluid build-up in the lungs due to lung cancer or other lung diseases. Discuss other possible alternatives with your doctor. Some diuretic are safer than others.

No. 25 -- **Trimethoprim + Sulfamethoxazole** -- Used to treat a wide variety of infections, including ear infections, urinary tract infections, bronchitis, diarrhea and other problems.

Potential Dangers -- You must not take this drug if you are deficient in the B vitamin folic acid. Also causes allergic reaction in many people. Caution must be used with people who have liver or kidney problems. Must drink large glass of water with the drug to prevent problems with the kidneys. Infants under two months should not have the drug. Can cause nausea, vomiting and stomach upset in adults and children.

Possible alternatives -- Infections are best avoided by healthy living, and by developing a strong immune system through good diet and plenty of exercise. Garlic is said to have antibiotic properties, but is not nearly as strong as prescription preparations. People with serious infections should not assume garlic is a good substitute, although it may help with minor infections. Again, the best way to deal with infections is to prevent them from happening in the first place. That means a healthy diet, with daily adequate amounts of vitamins A, D, E, C, B complex, and the minerals calcium, chromium, copper, iron, magnesium, manganese, molybdenum, selenium, zinc and beta cerotine.

No. 26 -- **Cipro** -- Another drug to treat urinary tract infections and ear infections. Often seen as an alternative to the drug listed above in the No. 25 spot. But this drug is also used for sexually transmitted diseases, prostatitis, skin injections and various bone infections.

Potential Dangers -- Many reports have been made of severe or even fatal allergic reactions to this drug even after the first dose. Other less deadly, but still troubling allergic reactions can also occur. Should be avoided by people with seizure disorders.

Infections are best avoided by healthy living, and by developing a strong immune system through good diet and plenty of exercise. Garlic is said to have antibiotic properties, but is not nearly as strong as prescription preparations. People with serious infections should not assume garlic is a good substitute, although it may help with minor infections. Again, the best way to deal with infections is to prevent them from happening in the first place. That means a healthy diet, with daily adequate amounts of vitamins A, D, E, C, B complex, and the minerals calcium, chromium, copper, iron, magnesium, manganese, molybdenum, selenium, zinc and beta cerotine.

No. 27 -- **Prempro** -- This is another estrogen supplement drug, sometimes used in lieu of Premarin, the No. 1 drug on our list. The female hormone that occurs naturally in the human body. Prempro is prescribed for women experiencing menopause, osteoporosis, ovarian failure, breast cancer, prostate cancer in men, bleeding of the uterus, vaginal irritation, birth control and Turner's

Syndrome.

Potential Dangers: Has been associated with increased chances of getting cancer, especially endometrial cancer. Women who smoke while taking this drug greatly increase chance of cancer. Prempro can also cause vaginal bleeding, breast tenderness, pain in feet and legs, rapid weight gain, sudden severe headaches and more.

Possible substitutes -- If Prempro is taken, many doctors will combine it with progesterone, which has shown to reduce the risk of cancer. But a natural substance that provides natural estrogen is tofu -- made from soybeans. Tofu and other soybean-based foods can supply large amounts of natural estrogen if eaten every day, or almost every day.

No. 28 -- **K-Dur** -- This is a potassium supplement prescribed for a condition called hypokalemia, or low blood potassium levels. Potassium is one of the most vital elements of a healthy human body. Without it, electrical impulses could not flow through the body's nervous system properly. Potassium is also vital for proper kidney function. The heart and other muscles cannot function without it. Potassium also regulates how the body used proteins and carbohydrates. Doctors prescribe K-Dur in a variety of situations. For example, when a patient is taking a diuretic prescription drug, such as Lasik or Furosemide, they may deplete their natural levels of potassium.

Potential Dangers -- This drug should be closely monitored by a physician. It is known to cause ulcers in the stomach and bowels. It can also lead to compression of the esophagus making it difficult or impossible to swallow solid foods. People taking this drug should avoid sun exposure, or risk side-effects. People with kidney or heart disease can be sickened or killed by K-Dur. Many people on K-Dur experience vomiting and dizziness. Do not use K-Dur with many salt substitutes, because they also contain potassium.

Possible substitutes -- Potassium can be obtained in many natural foods, and studies have shown that these natural sources of potassium can do a great job in replacing the need for K-Dur. Foods especially good and rich in potassium include bananas, apricots, acorn squash, avocados, beans, beef, broccoli, brussels sprouts, butternut squash, cantaloupe, chicken, collard greens, dates, fish, ham, kidney beans, lentils, orange juice, potatoes with skin, prunes, raisins, shellfish, spinach, split peas, turkey, veal, yogurt, white navy beans, watermelon and zucchini.

29 -- **Glucophage** -- This is a drug prescribed for people with diabetes mellitus. It is most often a second choice to treat diabetes. Glucophage is prescribed when other more popular diabetes drugs fail to respond in some patients.

Potential Dangers -- This drug is dangerous for people with heart or kidney conditions. It also produced negative allergic reactions in some people. The most common side effects are vomiting, diarrhea, nausea, abdominal bloating, stomach gas and loss of appetite, which can be an especially bad problem for diabetics who need to monitor their food intake with extreme care. About 3 in every 100 people who use Glucophage can experience an unpleasant metallic taste in the mouth, although it usually goes away without further treatment needed. About 9% of people on this drug also develop low levels of vitamin B-12. Should not be taken with alcohol.

Possible alternatives -- Diabetic, especially people with a severe case have few alternatives than to take one prescription drug of another. Still, patients can lessen the amount of drugs they need if they adopt lifestyles and diets that promote optimum health. That means a high fiber diet rich in fruits and vegetables and small amounts of meat. It also means avoiding alcohol and other food which contribute to problems.

No. 30 -- **Cephalexin** -- This is a popular antibiotic similar to penicillin. It is used to treat infections.

Potential Dangers -- Many people are allergic to this drug. The most common reactions is hives or an all-over-the-body rash. In the most serious cases death can result. Most common side effects are stomach pain and gas. Headaches, dizziness and nausea are also possible.

Possible alternatives -- Infections are best avoided by healthy living, and by developing a strong immune system through good diet and plenty of exercise. Garlic is said to have antibiotic properties, but is not nearly as strong as prescription preparations. People with serious infections should not assume garlic is a good substitute, although it may help with minor infections. Again, the best way to deal with infections is to prevent them from happening in the first place. That means a healthy diet, with daily adequate amounts of vitamins A, D, E, C, B complex, and the minerals calcium, chromium, copper, iron, magnesium, manganese, molybdenum, selenium, zinc and beta cerotine.

No. 31 -- **Acetaminophen with codeine** -- Most commonly called Tylenol-3, this is a widely prescribed pain killer for minor to moderate pain.

Potential Dangers -- This is a highly addictive drug. Codeine is an opiate, meaning it is originally designed after the opium drug. Also, because this drug contain Tylenol, it is potentially danger to the liver. The problem is two-fold -- many people become addicted to the codeine in this drug, which tempts them to take large doses of Tylenol. Taking more than 1,000 milligrams of Tylenol per day can cause serious liver damage or death.

Possible alternatives -- There are many alternatives for dealing with pain, including milder over-the-counter drugs such as plain Tylenol and aspirin. There is also accupunture, message, meditation and biofeedback. There are many alternative herbal remedies. For example, feverfew is indicated for headaches. If you have pain, seek to deal with it naturally before you consider this risk of getting addicted to this very tricky medication.

No. 32 -- **Amoxicillin trihydrate** -- This is another commonly used antibiotic very similar to penicillin. It is used to treat infections and infectious diseases.

Potential dangers -- Biggest danger is allergic reaction, which can be minor, or a serious as death. This drug can counter the effects of oral contraceptives. If you don't want to get pregnant, don't take this drug while you are on the pill. Allergic reactions are made stronger by beta-blockers. May increase the effect of blood thinners, such as aspirin. If you take the drug with fruit juice or a carbonated beverage, it will not be effective. Not recommended for women best feeding, although the risk is small.

Possible alternatives -- Best way to deal with infections is to avoid them in the first place. That means developing a healthy immune system with a healthy diet, regular exercise and vitamin rich diet that includes high amounts of fruits and vegetables. Garlic in known to have antibiotic properties. Taking garlic on a daily basis may keep you from serious infection, but is not guaranteed.

No. 33 -- **Hytrin** -- This is a drug used to treat high blood pressure. It is in a class of drugs called Alpha Blockers.

Potential Dangers -- Can cause dizziness and fainting. The first dose is especially likely to cause this effect. Many people are allergic to alpha blockers. It may also reduce both red and white blood cell counts. Many people experience headaches when taking this drug.

Possible alternatives -- Garlic is known to lower blood pressure and protect against heart disease. Also, many forms of meditation, yoga and breathing exercises lower blood pressure. A low fat diet or vegetarian diet can help lower blood pressure. Reduce stressful situations in life and find ways to be happy. See extensive advice listed in No. 18 of this chapter.

No. 34 -- **Darvon (Propoxyphen-N with APAP)** -- This is a fairly powerful narcotic pain reliever, most commonly called Darvon.

Potential Dangers -- Very addictive and causes many people to overdose. More than 1,000 death result every year as the result of overdosing. When this drug was introduced in 1957 by Eli Lilly, the makers of Prozac. Even though studies show that this drug is no more effective than aspirin, it is many time more dangerous. It makes little sense to use this drug over safer drugs like aspirin and Tylenol.

Possible alternatives -- There are many alternatives for dealing with pain, including milder over-the-counter drugs such as plain Tylenol and aspirin. There is also accupunture, message, meditation and biofeedback. There are many alternative herbal remedies. For example, feverfew is indicated for headaches. If you have pain, seek to deal with it naturally before you consider this risk of getting addicted to this potentially very dangerous medication.

No. 35 -- **Pravachol** -- Another of the drugs in the Statin class, used for lowering cholesterol. Similar to Zocor, Lipitor and Baycol, the deadliest of the statins. See chapter in this book devoted to Baycol and the other statins.

Potential Dangers -- While this drug was initially believed to be extremely safe, the most recent evidence is that it has some serious potential dangers, and its use could result in death. Statins were recently discovered to have caused at least 100 deaths in the U.S. alone. They can cause muscle tissue to dissolve and leach into the blood stream. The dead muscle cells then infect the kidneys and cause serious illness or death. Pravachol has also been strongly linked to cancer. In tests, it easily caused cancer in rats and mice, and almost certainly could cause cancer in humans. While rats were given Pravachol for only two years and developed cancer, humans take it for up to 10 years.

Possible alternatives -- The best way to reduce cholesterol in just about all people is to cut down on fatty foods and start a good exercise program. Stay away from greasy meats and favor fruits and vegetables. Stop smoking. Avoid coffee and caffeine. Also, fish oil and garlic supplements are known cholesterol fighters. They are many times safer if not overused. It makes little sense to rely on a possibly very dangerous drug like Zocor when so many goods alternatives are available.

No. 36 -- **Ultram** -- This is a nonnarcotic pain reliever. Introduced by the makers of Prozac in 1995, this painkiller was touted as being better and safer than aspirin.

Potential Dangers -- Because it was not a narcotic, Ultram it was deemed free of addiction problems. It was rushed through the FDA approval process, and deemed extremely safe and effective. But later Johnson & Johnson studied the drug and determined that the drug was actually extremely addictive. Stopping use of the drug can be very difficult. Also, the drug is known to cause seizures. Other side effects are dizziness, nausea, sweating, constipation, tiredness and itching. Large doses can cause inability to breath. There are other side effects as well.

Possible alternatives -- There are many alternatives for dealing with pain, including milder over-the-counter drugs such as plain Tylenol and aspirin. There is also accupunture, message, meditation and biofeedback. There are many alternative herbal remedies. For example, feverfew is indicated for headaches. If you have pain, seek to deal with it naturally before you consider this risk of getting addicted to this very tricky medication.

No. 37 -- **Veetids** -- This is a penicillin antibiotic. It is used to treat infections and infectious diseases.

Potential dangers -- Biggest danger is allergic reaction, which can be minor, or a serious as death. This drug can counter the effects of oral contraceptives. If you don't want to get pregnant, don't take this drug while you are on the pill. Allergic reactions are made stronger by beta-blockers. May increase the effect of blood thinners, such as aspirin. If you take the drug with fruit juice or a carbonated beverage, it will not be effective. Not recommended for women best feeding, although the risk is small.

Possible alternatives -- Best way to deal with infections is to avoid them in the first place. That means developing a healthy immune system with a healthy diet, regular exercise and vitamin rich diet that includes high amounts of fruits and vegetables. Garlic in known to have antibiotic properties. Taking garlic on a daily basis may keep you from serious infection, but is not guaranteed.

No. 38 -- **Dilantin** -- An antiseizure medication most often prescribed to people with epilepsy. It is the most prescribed of all the antiseizure drugs. Also sometimes prescribed for the prevention of migraine headaches.

Potential Dangers -- Has been linked with causing cancer. Should not be used by people with low blood pressure or slow heart rate. Poses problems for people with liver disease. Can lower white blood cell count and cause rashes in some individuals. Some people experience rapid growth of the gums, slurred speech, mental confusion, uncontrolled movement of the eyes, dizziness, insomnia, nervousness, uncontrollable twitching, double vision tiredness, irritability and depression.

Possible alternatives -- Especially for people with severe cases of epilepsy, there are probably few good alternatives to modern drugs. There are a variety of other antiseizure medication which some people may tolerate better than Dilantin. However, there is good evidence that a supplement of 250 IU of vitamin E per day may drastically reduce the chances of having a seizure. Also, a healthy lifestyle, plenty of exercise and a superior diet will help reduce the likelihood of seizures, as will elimination of stress in daily life. Also, meditation and accupuncture may be of enormous benefit and may drastically reduce the need for antiseizure medications.

No. 39 -- **Propacet 100** -- This is a pain killer very similar to Darvon. Unlike Darvon, it also contains acetaminophen, or Tylenol.

Potential Dangers -- Very addictive and causes many people to overdose. Many deaths result every year as the result of overdosing. Even though studies show that this drug is no more effective than aspirin or Tylenol, it is many time more dangerous. It makes little sense to use this drug over safer drugs such as plain aspirin and plain Tylenol.

Possible alternatives -- There are many alternatives for dealing with pain, including milder over-the-counter drugs, such as plain Tylenol and aspirin. There is also accupunture, message, meditation and biofeedback. There are many alternative herbal remedies. For example, feverfew is indicated for headaches. If you have pain, seek to deal with it naturally before you consider this risk of getting addicted to this potentially very dangerous medication.

No. 40 -- **Mevacor** -- Another of the recently enormously popular statins drugs that reduce cholesterol. See chapter in this book devoted to the dangers of these drugs.

While this drug was initially believed to be extremely safe, the most recent evidence is that it has some serious potential dangers, and its use could result in death. Statins were recently discovered to have caused at least 100 deaths in the U.S. alone. They can cause muscle tissue to dissolve and leach into the blood stream. The dead muscle cells then infect the kidneys and cause serious illness or death. This drug may cause cancer. In tests, it easily caused cancer in rats and mice, and almost certainly could cause cancer in humans. While rats were given Mevacor for only two years and developed cancer, humans take it for up to 10 years.

Possible alternatives -- The best way to reduce cholesterol in just about all people is to cut down on fatty foods and start a good exercise program. Stay away from greasy meats and favor fruits and vegetables. Stop smoking. Avoid coffee and caffeine. Also, fish oil and garlic supplements are known cholesterol fighters. They are many times safer if not overused. It makes little sense to rely on a possibly very dangerous drug like Zocor when so many goods alternatives are available.

No. 41 -- **Pepcid** -- Used to treat ulcers and heartburn. Was once only available by prescription, but now can be bought over the counter without a doctor's prescription.

Potential Dangers -- Probably pretty safe, but not without its problems. Can cause headaches, dizziness, diarrhea and constipation. Also can give the user a false sense that they do not have to worry about ulcers or stomach bleeding and can encourage people to assume bad habits, such as smoking and eating poor, greasy foods.

Possible alternatives -- Heartburn has little or nothing to do with your heart. The problem is with the door between your esophagus and stomach. As you know, your stomach contains powerful acids used to digest foods. When the doorway to the stomach — called the esophageal sphincter — fails to close properly, it lets acid from the stomach back up into your esophagus. While your stomach is designed for digestive acids, your esophagus is not, and the result is a powerful burning sensation.

So how do you get the doorway to close properly? Well, don't do things that will weaken the esophageal sphincter, and those things are:

(a) Smoking. Once again, the Demon Weed finds a new way to create trouble in your life. Smoking cigarettes weakens the esophageal sphincter considerably. Don't complain about heartburn if you're not trying to curb your smoking. Without stopping, you don't have much chance of booting the problem.

(b) No napping. It seems almost natural to take a nap after a big meal, but that makes gravity work against you. Acid will more easily travel upward into your esophagus if your are horizontal. Let your food digest a bit before you lie down.

(c) No bedtime snacks. Your stomach can produce acid for up to seven hours after you eat. If you eat just before you go to bed, you may be setting yourself up for a late-night acid or heartburn attack that will ruin your sleep, and thus the following day. Skip the bedtime snack if you are prone to heartburn.

(c) Avoid Stress. Perhaps the No. 1 cause of heartburn behind coffee and cigarettes is stress and anxiety. Stress, fear and anxiety gets the acid factory in your stomach pumping. Take a time out, or a meditation break to calm yourself and your body down. (See headings under "Meditation", "Stress").

(d) Coffee, chocolate and caffeine. Avoid them all. Make no doubt about it — they are all major, we repeat MAJOR, causes of heartburn. (See heading under "Three Terrible C's").

What will help

(a) Milk, antacids, bicarbonate of soda or soda crackers. All of these are well known counter-agents of heartburn and they usually work, so why not try them?

(b) Lose weight. A common contributor to heartburn is obesity.

Losing weight will be good for your total health, so do it for more than easing heartburn.

(c) Eat smaller meals more often. Rather than big honking meals that distend your belly and make you waddle like a duck, easing food into your stomach a little at a time all day will give your stomach a chance to digest, and will not force food upwards to make room in limited space.

Persistent heartburn

Many TV commercials now warn about the dangers of persistent heartburn, while at the same time pushing their over-the-counter products as the solution. This makes little sense. If you have long-term, recurring heartburn, and if you need to keep taking over-the-counter medicine day after day, then you probably should see a doctor. Remember, frequent heartburn can lead to more serious problems, such as ulcers, gastritis (inflammation of the stomach wall), stomach cancer and other problems. Use your common sense. Deal with it.

No. 42 -- **Zithromax** -- This is an antibiotic, called a Marcolide antibiotic. It is used to treat upper respiratory tract infections, skin infections and sexually transmitted diseases. It is also used to treat a variety of other infectious conditions.

Potential dangers -- Like its cousin penicillin, it can cause severe allergic reactions in some people. Should not be taken by people with liver disease or kidney problems. Another disease associated with this drug is colitis, which is inflammation of the bowels.

Possible alternatives -- Best way to deal with infections is to avoid them in the first place. That means developing a healthy immune system with a healthy diet, regular exercise and vitamin rich diet that includes high amounts of fruits and vegetables. Garlic in known to have antibiotic properties. Taking garlic on a daily basis may keep you from serious infection, but is not guaranteed. Also, avoid risky behavior, such as that which can expose you to sexually transmitted diseases. The best way to fight an infection of this kind is to never get it.

No. 43 -- **Humulin** -- This is insulin for diabetics who cannot control their condition with diet alone.

Potential Dangers -- Patient must be very careful to take exact dosage or risk serious health problems, including coma and death. Patient should avoid alcohol and stay on carefully controlled diet.

Possible alternatives -- There are no alternatives. But diabetics can dramatically improve their conditions by maintaining careful diets and checking blood sugar often. A healthy lifestyle that includes avoiding alcohol and smoking will greatly improve general health and reduce problems associated with diabetes.

No. 44 -- **Ambien** -- This a sedative prescribed for sleeping problems. It's a sleeping pill.

Potential Dangers -- This drug should never be taken for longer than 10 days. You may find if difficult to ever fall asleep normally again. Sleep problems usually have an underlying cause, whether due to disease or psychological anxiety. It is better to get to the root of the problem, rather than rely on a drug like this to varnish over the problem over a long period.

Possible alternatives -- There are many herbal preparations that aid sleep. Vitamin B-6 deficiency can cause insomnia, so increasing your intake of this vitamin can aid sleep. Vitamin B-12 also helps. It's probably best to take a B-Complex supplement to make sure you are getting all the B-vitamins you need on a daily basis. Do not megadose on vitamin B. Trace minerals are also extremely important to sleep. People low in copper, for example, often have trouble sleeping. A high magnesium and low-aluminum diet also aid sleep. Calcium interacts with magnesium to make sleep come more easily and naturally. Another excellent natural substance for aiding sleep is called tryptophan. This is an amino acid found in all protein-rich foods. Turkey is an excellent source of tryptophan. Warm milk has long been associated with helping people get to sleep, and it probably works. Poor sleep is most often the result of the intake of our most popular daily vices -- caffeine, alcohol and sugar. Cut down drastically on these substances, and your sleep patterns may soon become blissfully normal. One last substance associated with disturbing sleep is MSG, or monosodium glutamate. This can be found in many canned and/or processed foods. Many Chinese foods are associated with high MSG content. Check with your favorite Chinese restaurant to see if they use high amounts of MSG in their foods. If they do, avoid them. Reducing daily stress, such as stress at work or in relationship is a major factor in getting a good night's sleep. Taking up a calming practice, such as meditation or a daily good exercise workout can work wonders in helping people sleep peacefully and normally.

No. 45 -- **Prinivil** -- This drug is used to treat high blood pressure, congestive heart failure and improving survival after heart attack. It is in a class of drugs called ACE inhibitors.

Potential Dangers -- Is known to cause kidney problems. Can cause headaches, dizziness, fatigue, nausea, diarrhea and chronic cough. Can also swell the tongue and hinder breathing. Is probably more dangerous for seniors. Has been associated with stroke in rare cases, and also impotence.

Possible alternatives -- Garlic is known to lower blood pressure and protect against heart disease. Also, many forms of meditation, yoga and breathing exercises lower blood pressure. A low fat diet or vegetarian diet can help lower blood pressure. Reduce stressful situations in life and find ways to be happy.

No. 46 -- **Relafen** -- This is a nonsteroidal anti-inflammatory drug used to treat arthritis. Among a class of drugs known as NSAIDS. They reduce pain and inflammation.

Potential dangers - This drug and all NSAIDS are extremely controversial and associated with dozens of dangers, but mostly with causing serious damage to the stomach. As many as 700,000 may be hospitalized every year because of severe stomach or gastrointestinal bleeding caused by these drugs.

Possible alternatives -- There are many nondrug and natural alternatives for treating arthritis. One of the most effective natural treatments may be fish oil, or more specifically omega-3 fatty acids. This substance is found in many variety of fish, but especially salmon, mackerel, sardines and herring. You can also buy omega-3 in capsule form and take it as a daily supplement if you don't like to eat fish. It is believed, however, that getting this oil directly from the fish is the better way. Arthritis is strongly linked to poor diets. If you improve your diet in a general sense, you may see an improvement in your condition. Getting enough vitamin D and calcium is essential. Switching to a vegetarian diet greatly improves and even cures arthritis is some people. Eliminating certain foods may also help, especiacally polyunsaturated vegetable oils, including corn oil, sesame, sunflower, and safflower. Eliminating margarine is a good idea, too. Many herbal remedies are believed to be effective in treating arthritis, including evening-primrose oil, ginger, turmeric and willow bark. Acupuncture has been remarkably successful for many arthritics.

More arthritis advice: Your arthritis may have a lot to do with a poor diet, and a proliferation of yeast cells in your digestive system. Yeast cells occur naturally in your intestinal tract, but sometimes antibiotic drugs, a diet of too many sweets, breads, meats and mold-bearing foods can produce an overpopulation of yeast cells in your body. The result is a lot of toxic secretions by the cells into your bloodstream, resulting in many adverse effects, including arthritis.

One of the best natural "yeast cell killers" is garlic. If you dramatically increase your garlic intake — say by one or two cloves per day — you may notice beneficial effects within a couple of weeks. You can also buy easy to take garlic supplements at any drug store or supermarket.

Garlic, in general, has long been used for its beneficial effects on inflammation and arthritis. Give garlic a try. At worst, it a nutritional food that will be a positive supplement to your overall diet.

Give up sweets

For one thing, sweets are a primary food for yeast cells. Avoiding sweets, breads (which contain yeast) too much meat and mold-bearing foods will help cleans your body of toxics and starve yeast cells. Sweets in general, especially white sugar, have long been suspects in aggravating arthritis. Even if it does not help your arthritis, giving up sweets will be beneficial for many other reasons, from weight control to improving your overall diet.

Give up coffee

Coffee is one of the worst substances for people with arthritis. First, it has a high level of acidity which can help break down cartilage in joints and contribute to the advancement of arthritis. Caffeine contributes to stress and nervousness — both major culprits in increasing the pain and progress of arthritis. There are also many other oils and substances in coffee that are believed to worsen arthritis symptoms. In short, if you have arthritis, coffee is one of the worst things you can give it.

Try a low-fat diet

The connection between diet and arthritis has long been controversial. For many years The Arthritis Foundation has dismissed any connection between diet and arthritis. One of the Foundations pamphlet reads: "The possible relationship between diet and arthritis has been thoroughly and scientifically studied ... the simple proven fact is that no food has anything to do with causing arthritis and no food is effective in treating it."

But we're sorry, Arthritis Foundation — your are clearly wrong about this one. The fact is, many people have discovered real relief by switching to a diet low in fat, and high in fiber and vitamin. According to the book, Arthritis Relief, by Jean Wallace, many new studies show that a low-fat diet can have a significant effect on relieving arthritis symptoms.

Doctors at the University of Florida, for example, have found that certain foods, such as dairy products and shrimp, trigger flair-ups in a small amount of sensitive people. An improved, leaner diet with little or no meat has helped a large number of people to significantly reduce inflammation, and relieve the fatigue associated with arthritis. Your really owe it to yourself to try a low-fat diet for several months. You have nothing to lose but a lot of fat and cholesterol, and you may gain a upper hand against the persistent and insidious disease of arthritis.

Avoid milk

Still on the diet note, a lot evidence suggests that milk may be the culprit behind many people's affliction of rheumatoid arthritis. This includes food such as cookies and cakes, which may contain milk as an ingredient. Stop drinking milk for a couple of months and see what happens.

Eat more fish

There is now solid evidence that certain fish oils may

suppress symptoms of arthritis. The fish oil identified with helping arthritis is omega-3, and is found in freshwater fish, especially salmon. Omega-3 supplements are also available in health food stores, but taking these is less effective and less desirable than getting your omega-3 directly from the source. Fish oil tablets may cause belching or loose stools.

Some other allergy?

Your arthritis may be the result of another food entirely. Everyone is different, and you may have a specific allergy to a specific food. Identifying such a food is not easy. Perhaps the best idea is to keep a journal of your symptoms, keeping a close eye on your level of pain and inflammation, and then trying to match it up with something you have eaten recently. Once you think you have found something that makes your pain worse, avoid that food for several weeks, then try it again in as a test. If your body reacts negatively, then you may have isolated something that is giving you trouble.

Give these natural herbs a try

All of these herbs and special preparations have been identified with helping or healing arthritis. You can find all of these herbs in your health food store. Search them out and try them out for at least three months:

Devil's Claw	Tumeric
Bilberry	Hawthorne
Bromelain	Hawthrone Berry
Burdock Root	Yucca Powder
Sarsaparilla Root	Ginger Root
Willow Bark	Ginseng

Eat a lot more of these foods

Pineapple	Pineapple juice
Garlic	Brazil nuts
Herring	Salmon
Onions	Broccoli

No. 47 -- **Atrovent** -- This is a drug used to treat bronchospasm that is related to lung diseases, such as bronchitis and emphysema. It is also prescribed for allergies and the common cold.

Potential Dangers -- Can cause moderate to sever allergic reactions in many people. Should not be used by people with prostate problems, glaucoma or bladder obstruction. This drug is relatively safe and has few and mild side effects. The most common side effects are nervousness, dizziness, headache, nausea, upset stomach, blurred vision, sensitivity to bright light, dry mouth, throat irritation, cough, worsening of symptoms it is supposed to treat, rash, heart palpitations and mouth irritation.

Possible alternatives -- Maintaining proper amounts of vitamin A and beta-carotene are essential for healthy lungs and the prevention of lung disorders. Vitamin E supplements can also prevent lung problems. Other important vitamins are the B's and vitamin C. Inadequate amounts of copper in the human body can lead to many and frequent problems with the lungs. Taking a selenium supplement is helpful. Optimal magnesium intake might prevent or treat a number of lung disorders that Atrovent is used to treat. Avoid tobacco smoke and other environmental pollutants to keep the lungs healthy and free of bronchitis or emphysema.

No. 48 -- **Ibuprofin** -- A very common drug also sold as Advil, Nuprin, Midol, Motrin Children's Advil and many more. Can be bought over-the-counter or in prescription strength from a doctor. It is an NSAID. It is used to treat inflammation and pain, including headaches, PMS and arthritis.

Potential Dangers -- NSAIDS are among the most controversial of all drugs. This drug and all NSAIDS are associated with dozens of dangers, but mostly with causing serious damage to the stomach. As many as 700,000 may be hospitalized every year because of severe stomach or gastrointestinal bleeding caused by these drugs.

Possible alternatives -- Alternatives depends on what you plan to use Ibuprofin for. Arthritics have a number of options, as outlined in No. 46. Women suffering PMS have dozens of alternatives, all of them natural and much safer. PMS is made worse by a lack of exercise, a diet high in fat and sugar and high consumption of caffeine and alcohol. Avoid these and avoid PMS. Also contributing to PMS is stress, poor diet, genetic factors and environment. Supplements that will help PMS include vitamin E, B-6, magnesium, calcium and manganese. Other pain relief, such as for headaches, can be obtained by accupuncture, meditation and healthy diet.

No. 49 -- **Alprazolem** -- Most commonly known as Xanax. Used treat anxiety, tension, fatigue and agitation.

Potential Dangers -- This is one of the most controversial, and possible one of the most addictive drugs ever made. People taking this drug have also become suicidal, gone insane or have become violent. Withdrawal from the drug is extremely difficult. Many people require hospitalization just to get off Xanax.

Possible alternatives -- Taking this drug should only be for extreme cases. Most people should deal with anxiety, tension and fatigue in natural ways, such as getting rid of a high stress job, fixing or getting out of bad relationships, talk therapy, meditation or an overall change of lifestyle. A relaxing daily or weekly massage, reflexology treatment or even daily vigorous exercise can be ten times more effective than Xanax. Adopting a spiritual practice of choice and a more quiet, sane lifestyle is the perfect substitute for trying to fix problems like anxiety, stress and fatigue with a powerful pill that can end up making you an addict, insane or dead.

No. 50 -- **Accupril** -- An ACE inhibitor, this drug is prescribed for high blood pressure and congestive heart failure.

Potential Dangers -- Causes allergic reactions in many patients. Should not be taken by people with low blood pressure. It may decrease white blood cell count leaving the patient more susceptible to infections. Most common side effects are dizziness, tiredness, headache and chronic cough. This drug is also affected by a high fat food diet. Doctors recommend it be taken on an empty stomach.

Possible alternatives -- Garlic is known to lower blood pressure and protect against heart disease. Also, many forms of meditation, yoga and breathing exercises lower blood pressure. A low fat diet or vegetarian diet can help lower blood pressure. Reduce stressful situations in life and find ways to be happy.

OTHER NOTABLE DRUGS -- AND LATE BREAKING WARNINGS!

VIAGRA -- This is a very high profile drug used to treat impotency, or male erectile dysfunction. in males. Billed as one of the first truly effective male sex enhancers, Viagra has sold briskly in all world markets.

THE DANGERS OF VIAGRA

Because sexual activity involves an increase in cardiac work and myocardial oxygen demand the FDA advises doctors to consider the cardiac status of patients who may receive Viagra.

The FDA also advises that Viagra NOT to prescribed to

patients who take organic nitrates in any form, regardless of frequency.

VIAGRA SHOULD NOT BE TAKEN BY MEN WHO: Combine a nitrate and Viagra at home. This can lead to severe hypotensiveness The nitrate contraindication cannot be stressed enough!

ALSO IMPORTANT: Men with no previous history of angina and who takes Viagra, can develop an anginal episode, or heart attack!

This is important to know because such a patient could be brought to an Emergency Department while still having chest pain, where a short-acting nitrate may routinely be administered to treat this. This could make the situation worse, not better!

Here is a list of drugs that are **ORGANIC NITRATES AND SHOULD NOT BE COMBINED WITH VIAGRA:**

Nitroglycerin

Deponit
Minitran
Nitrek
Nitro-Bid
Nitrocine
Nitro-Derm
Nitro Disc
Nitro-Dur
Nitrogard
Nitroglycerin
Nitroglycerin T/R
Nitroglyn
Nitrol Ointment
Nitrolan

Nitrolingual Spray
Nitrong
Nitropar
Nitropress
Nitroprex
Nitro S.A.
Nitrospan
Nitrostat
Nitro-Trans System
Nitro Transdermal
Nitro-Time
Transderm-Nitro
Tridil

Isosorbide Mononitrate

Imdur
ISMO
Isosorbide Mononitrate
Monoket

Isosorbide Nitrate

Dilatrate-SR
Iso-bid
Isordil
Isordil Tembids
Isosorbide Dinitrate
Isosorbide Dinitrate LA
Sorbitrate
Sorbitrate SA

Pentaerythritol Tetranitrate

Peritrate
Peritrate SA

Erythrityl Tetranitrate

Cardilate

Isosorbide Dinitrate/Phenobarbital

Isordil w/PB

Illicit Substances Containing Organic Nitrates

Such as, amyl nitrate or nitrite (It is known that amyl nitrate or nitrite is sometimes abused. In abused situations, amyl nitrate or nitrite may be known by various names, including "poppers.")

VIAGRA ALTERNATIVES:

Viagra is a controversial drugs. Some studies even conclude that Viagra does not work at all. So why do so many men report great results? It may be the placebo effect. Because men "think" they have received an erection enhancer, they get around the mental block which is at the root of the problem.

There are also some natural alternatives to Viagra. Let's talk about them.

But many people believe that certain substances are aphrodisiacs. Perhaps the most common in ginseng, which is especially popular in Oriental countries and cultures. And there may be something to, especially for females. A daily dose of ginseng extract, or ginseng tea is known to increase the level of testosterone in males. Testosterone of course is the "male hormone" and having a higher level of it may increase a man's libido and stamina in sexual activity.

Other more exotic substances are frequently sought for their purported aphrodisiacal properties, notable, powdered rhinoceros horns. In fact, the rhinoceros is being hunted to extinction because the demand for their horns is so high in China that many people are willing to take the great risk or poaching rhinos.

Like ginseng, however, powdered rhino horn is probably not an aphrodisiac.

But to say there are no aphrodisiac is not entirely true either. Several drugs, for example, clearly work with the human body chemistry to stimulate sexual function. The prescription drug bromocriptine (brand name is Parlodel) is very effective in reversing male impotency, and has been shown to increase libido by 80 percent in both males and females. Bromocriptine has also been know to return post-menopausal women to regular menstrual cycles, even women in their 60s and 70s!

Research has clearly shown that certain vitamins play an important role in increasing and enhancing sexuality. These foods may not be "love potions" or aphrodisiacs per say, but they do help along the chemicals in your brain — called neurotransmitters — which are needed for healthy sexual functioning.

Vitamin B-5 (also known as calcium pantothenate) may be able to increase your sexual stamina is you take it with lecithin and choline, both common items you can purchase in health food stores.

Another B vitamin, Niacin, or Vitamin B-6 plays an extremely important role in attaining orgasm. A chemical in your body called histamine, which has many functions, is closely associated with orgasm release. An amino acid called histidine in your body is converted into histamine by niacin. Niancin causes the release of histimine — which produces the flushed itching feeling often associated with orgasm.

Taking niacin supplements about a half hour or so before

having sex may assist in your ability to have an orgasm. Also, making sure you are getting enough niacin in your diet may help insure you have the ability to have an orgasm whenever you want to.

These foods are high in niacin, and therefore, may help sexual function:

Tuna (water packed)	mackerel
chicken breast	pink salmon
veal rump roast	Kaboom (cereal)
turkey breast	Product 19 (cereal)
cod	crabmeat
lamb	Quaker Instant Oatmeal

THE MOST IMPORTANT SEXUAL ORGAN IN THE BODY - - THE BRAIN!

Most people think the penis or the vagina is the center of sexual problems, but what sends signals to and from these organs? The brain! More often than not, this is where the cure for sexual dysfunction can be found. Thus, we urge anyone considering Viagra to first consider nondrug therapies that deal with the many potential mental blocks to proper sexual activity.

RITALIN -- THE CHILD'S DRUG

Ratalin is a drug most often prescribed to children who are diagnosed with Attention Deficit Disorder, or ADD. Interestingly, Ritalin is actually a brain stimulant, and speeds up the activity of the brain. So why does it make hyperactive children calm down? It is not clearly understood. Even the drug company that makes Ratlin says: "The mode of action in man is not completely understood. Ritalin presumably activates the brain stem arousal system and cortex."

AFFECTS UNKNOWN?

And this is exactly what is scary about Ritalin. Nobody is quite sure about just how it works -- yet people are willing to give it to their own children by the millions! Today, about 10 percent of all school-age children take Ritalin daily. This is truly a scary situation, ripe for disaster.

While we don't know how Ritalin works, we do know that it has irreversible side effects. It can cause a form of brain damage known as Touette's Syndrome. This diseases is characterized by tics, twitches, and abnormal sounds and movements from the child. Sometimes, these sounds and movements are truly bizarre, including uncontrolled urge to swear, scream, grunt, growl, and more.

Many times, this brain disease has continued in children even after they stopped taking Ritalin. Other side effects include loss of appetite, insomnia, and stomach problems.

RITALIN ABUSE AND ADDICTION

But Ritalin has another serious problems. Many drug addicts have discovered that by crushing Ritalin tablets into a powder and snorting it, they get an affect far better than that of cocaine. As of today, thousands of people are addicted to Ritalin. They began by using it as a recreational drug, only to find out that after just one or two snorts, stopping seems all but impossible. Naturally, many children are opting to experiment by crushing and snorting their own pills -- so instead of calming down, they're becoming dangerous, hyperactive drug freaks. Many parents are also turning on with Ritalin, snitching their children's medications for their own recreational use.

Finally, once a child is put on Ritalin, when and how do they get off? It's a good question, and the answer may be: "never."

Parents considering putting their children on Ritalin should consider the fact that such a decision may have life-long consequences. Those who try to stop using Ritalin will almost certainly face horrible withdrawal symptoms that may take months of hospitalization to take care off -- if they don't die in the process.

Fortunately, there are many nondrug alternatives for the problem of hyperactive children, including behavior modification therapy, a rigidly structured environment and special education scenarios. If these don't seem like a lot of fun, think about the alternative -- a lifetime of addiction to a powerful brain stimulant that may last forever.

Tylenol-3

Tylenol is the brand name for acetaminophen, but you can by it under dozens of other names, including it's generic name. But Tylenol can also be combined with the opiate codeine. There are several different prepartions, and they are usually delineated by numbers according to strength. Tylenol-1, for example, contains only 8 mg of codeine. This form of the drug can actaully be purchased without a prescription in some states, and throughout all of Canada without a prescription from a doctor.

Codeine is an extremely addictive drug, and thus Tylenol-3 tends to be a serious problem among drug addicts, or with hooking previously non-druging using people, turning them into addicts. Withdrawal from codeine addiction can be extremely painfully physically and also psychologically torturous. Part of the reason for this is that codeine is converted to morphine in the brain. This of course will result in a positive result in a drug test for the opiates. It is not known whether or not the drugs heroin, morphine or codeine can be separately determined on a drug test. In other words it isn't likely that the drug tester can determine which of the three above drugs you have taken, he just knows you've taken one or more of them.

The Tylenol-3 you get from a doctor contains 30 mg of codeine, and varying amounts of acetaminophen. There is also a Tylenol-4 with 60 mg of codeine. Codeine is a member of the drug class opiates. Opiates include all naturally occurring drugs with morphine-like effects such as codeine and all semi and fully synthetic drugs with morphine-like effects such as heroin and meperidine (Demerol). Codeine was first discovered as a natural constituent of opium in very small concentrations, in the range of 0.7% - 2.5% by weight. Most codeine found in pharmaceutical products today is synthetically produced via the methylation of morphine.

For the most part, codeine is used as a pain reliever, but is also used for the relief of a non-productive cough, and as a anti-diarrheal agent. 120mg of codeine administered SC (subcutaneously, injected under the skin) provides pain relief equal to 10mg of morphine administered by the same route. Doses used to relieve cough or diarrhea range from 5mg to 30mg. Codeine is absorbed quickly from the GI tract and it's first pass through the liver results in very little loss of the drug. This contrasts with morphine in which over 90% of the drug is metabolized in the first pass through the liver resulting in a considerable loss of potency when administered orally. This is why codeine is a common opiate in the relief of pain, the ease of oral administration.

Codeine can be taken by the patient or administered by a nurse or doctor in many ways. in many waysby many routes, this includes, SC, IM (intramuscularly), as an enema, and orally. Note, codeine can't be administered safely by IV (intravenously) injection as it can result in pulmonary edema (fluid in lungs), facial swelling and other life threatening complications.

Some common side effects from codeine include drowsiness, light-headedness, dry mouth, urinary retention (difficulty in urination), constipation and of course, euphoria. Adverse effects can include itchiness (common), confusion, nausea and vomiting. The nausea experienced with codeine is less common and less intense than that experienced with the stronger opiates such as morphine. A tip to all those using opiates, lying down does wonders to the nausea. If you ever experience nausea on opiates it is different than the commonly experienced nausea as it is more of a light-headed nausea. Lying down will almost always relieve the nausea in a couple minutes, which after you can attempt to stand up again.

The llethal dose for for the average person is about is 800m, so it is somewhat difficult to overdose on this drug. However, remember that acetaminophen is also a liver toxin, so even if you get far less than 800 mg of codeine, you will most likely getting enough of both of the drugs to do you in pretty easily. in the average person. Some sources say that as little as 250 to 400 mg of codeine can kill. Death from codeine, unlike most opiates, includes restlessness, seizures and eventually death from respiratory arrest.

The reason we include Tylenol-3 and Tylenol-4 here is its extreme popularity andits extreme addictiveness. Doctors, and dentists also, prescribe a lot of Tylenol-3 and Tylenol-4 every day. Many people report that they become addicted after just the very first dose. Tylenol-3 is one of the hottest "street drugs" around. Individual pills can sell for as much as $25 to $50 on the black market.

The drug is so popular because it produces an extremely pleasant, euphoric feeling. It's a true, blissful escape drug. For people with high stress or emotional problems, the escape that Tylenol-3 provides is highly desirable. That'why it's so easy to get hooked. Also, another major contributor to addiction is the fact that codeine's effect is quickly resisted by the body. That is, after the first several doses of Tylenol-3, it takes a bigger and bigger dose each time to get the same high one experienced the first time.

Many people who get Tylenol-3 or Tylenol-4 from the doctor

assume it is as safe as the ordinary Tylenol you can buy off the shelf. This is another reason why people develop addiction and ovesuse problems. The name Tylenol os one of the most trusted and well-known on the market. But you need to understand that the Tylenol you get from a doctor is actually a narcotic. If you are prescribed Tylenol-3 or -4 for pain, be it a toothache or a headache, use it only as prescribed. If you pain event ends, throw the remainder of the pills away.

Unfortunately, many people have ongoing or chronic pain. People who suffer frequent and persistent migraine headaches, for example, stand at great risk of addiction to drugs such as or like Tylenol-3. People with cancer or other pain-causing condition also risk addiction.

Perhaps the biggest tragedy of Tylenol-3 addiction is the fact that people with chronic pain who legitimately need the drug often have trouble convincing their doctor to prescribe it. Doctors are under close scrutiny by federal drug enforcement agencies to prescribe narcotics only when absolutely necessary. Thus, the tend to hold back when a painn-wracked patient is in great need.

You would be well advised to exhaust all other forms of nondrug-related pain therapy before you decide to risk taking Tylenol-3. Acupuncture, non-narcotic drug preparations, massage, acupressure and biofeedback are examples of pain relief possibilities. Hypnotism also works extremely well for a certain percentage of the population. Whatever the case, use caution when it comes to Tylenol-3 or Tylenol-4. It's not just ordinary Tylenol!

LATE BREAKING NEWS AND WARNINGS:

The Following are some late breaking warnings issued by the FDA and media sources just as this book was going to press:

Ultra Botanicals Recalls "MSM Eye Drops" and "MSM Eyes & Nasal Drops"

Ultra Botanicals, Inc. of Los Angeles is recalling all lots of its 1 ounce bottles of "MSM Eye Drops" and "MSM Eyes & Nasal Drops" due to potentially serious health risks associated wit bacterial contamination and the lack of evidence demonstrating the safety of MSM for use in the eyes or nose.

Samples analyzed by the Food and Drug Administration were found to contain Pseudomonas mendocina and Klebsiella pneumoniae, bacteria that in some case can cause sight-threatening injury.

The recalled "MSM Eye Drops" were distributed nationwide and sold in retail stores. The recalled "MSM Eyes & Nasal Drops" were sold directly to consumers.

Both products are manufactured in 1 ounce dropper bottles. "MSM Eye Drops" are labeled and sold under the Ultra Botanicals brand, while "MSM Eyes & Nasal Drops" were distributed under the All That's Natural brand.

To date, there have been no reports of injury in connection with these products. Individuals who have used these products and have experienced any adverse reactions are advised to contact their health care provider.

Consumers who have purchased 1-ounce bottles of "MSM Eye Drops" or "MSM Eyes & Nasal Drops" are urged to return them to the place of purchase for a full refund. Consumers with questions may contact the company at 1-800-357-7655.

POPULAR COLD REMEDIES THAT COULD KILL

The Food and Drug Administration advised consumers

Monday to avoid over-the-counter cold remedies and have appetite suppressants with a common alternative ingredient linked to increased stroke risk, and it called on drug companies to stop using the ingredient.

Consumers may still find the products in their drugstores for several months until the FDA rule, which in effect bans the Alka-Seltzer Plus ingredient's use in non-prescription remedies, is in cold remedies place.

Comtrex Flu Therapy & Fever Relief
Contac 12 Hour Cold Capsules
Coricidin D Cold Flu & Sinus
Dimetapp DM Cold & Cough Elixir
Robitussin CF

A Yale University study, which Day & Night found that phenylpropanolamine, or PPA, increased stroke risk in some users, spurred an FDA advisory committee last month to conclude that the product is not safe.

The study is scheduled to appear Dec. 21 in The New England Journal of Medicine , but the journal took the unusual move of posting it on its Web site early because of "potential public health implications."

Americans consume 4.5 billion doses a year of non-prescription PPA, according to the FDA. An FDA reviewer told the advisory committee that products with PPA might be responsible for 200 to 500 hemorrhagic strokes (bleeding in the brain) each year in U.S. adults younger than 50.

The federal agency, concerned about alarming consumers, decided not to pull PPA products immediately from store shelves, says Charles Ganley, the top FDA official for over-the-counter drugs.

"It's a very rare occurrence," Ganley says of PPA-linked strokes. "The product's been marketed out there for many years. Taking those things into account, we didn't think it fell into that immediate-hazard category."

Still, Ganley says, the FDA felt it was important to alert consumers to the potential risk by issuing a public health warning.

In a statement, R. William Soller, director of science and technology at the Consumer Healthcare Products Association, a trade group, continued to defend the safety of PPA-containing products.

Companies are reviewing the FDA's action and will decide how to proceed, according to Soller's statement. Ganley says several drug makers contacted the FDA after the advisory committee meeting to discuss reformulating their products without PPA.

Though there are other compounds that could replace PPA in decongestants, it is the only approved over-the-counter appetite-suppressing drug.

FDA WARNS AGAINST NATURE'S NUTRITION FORMULA ONE

The Food and Drug Administration is warning consumers not to purchase or consume Nature's Nutrition Formula One products labeled as containing Ma huang (ephedrine) and kola nut because the product poses a risk to consumers' health. The products are sold by Alliance U.S.A. of Richardson, Texas.

THE FDA has determined that the products can cause severe injury or death in some people who consume them. Nature's

Nutrition Formula One is labeled as a diet supplement and has been marketed with labeling purporting that it is useful for weight loss and energy enhancement. The potentially dangerous products can be identified by the listing of Ma huang and kola nut as ingredients and the appearance of either of the following usage statements on the label: "Adult Food Supplement Take 1 to 3 capsules at 10:00 AM & 3:00 PM," or "Adult food supplement: one to two capsules mid-morning and mid-afternoon."

FDA has received more than 100 reports of injuries and adverse reactions related to the product during the past year. Reported reactions range from serious, life-threatening conditions such as irregular heartbeat, heart attack, stroke, seizures, hepatitis and psychosis, to relatively minor and temporary conditions such as dizziness, headache and gastrointestinal distress. Several deaths have been associated with the product.

FDA and outside medical experts have determined that the products represent a threat to health because the combination of Ma huang, a source of ephedrine, and kola nut, a source of caffeine, can cause severe injury to people even under conditions of usual or recommended use. Ephedrine is an amphetamine-like chemical that acts as a stimulant in the body.

The FDA's warning is limited to versions of Nature's Nutrition Formula One that contain both Ma huang and kola nut. The company has advised FDA that it has reformulated its product to remove the kola nut. This warning does not apply to the reformulated version of the product.

Glossary

Addiction: A chronic, relapsing disease, characterized by compulsive drug seeking and use and by neurochemical and molecular changes in the brain.

Barbiturate: A type of central nervous system (CNS) depressant often prescribed to promote sleep.

Benzodiazepine: A type of CNS depressant prescribed to relieve anxiety; among the most widely prescribed medications, including Valium and Librium.

Buprenorphine: A new medication awaiting FDA approval for treatment of opioid addiction. It blocks the effects of opioids on the brain.

Central nervous system (CNS): The brain and spinal cord.

CNS depressants: A class of drugs that slow CNS function, some of which are used to treat anxiety and sleeping disorders; includes barbiturates and benzodiazepines.

Detoxification: A process that allows the body to rid itself of a drug while at the same time managing the individual's symptoms of withdrawal; often the first step in a drug treatment program.

Dopamine: A neurotransmitter present in regions of the brain that regulate movement, emotion, motivation, and feelings of pleasure.

LAAM (levo-alpha-acetyl-methadol): An approved medication for the treatment of opioid addiction, taken 3 to 4 times a week.

Methadone: A long-acting synthetic medication that is effective in treating opioid addiction.

Narcolepsy: A disorder characterized by uncontrollable episodes of deep sleep.

Norepinephrine: A neurotransmitter present in some areas of the brain and the adrenal glands; decreases smooth muscle contraction and increases heart rate; often released in response to low blood pressure or stress.

Opioids: Controlled drugs or narcotics most often prescribed for the management of pain; natural or synthetic chemicals based on opium's active component - morphine - that work by mimicking the actions of pain-relieving chemicals produced in the body.

Opiophobia: A health care provider's unfounded fear that patients will become physically dependent upon or addicted to opioids even when using them appropriately; can lead to the underprescribing of opioids for pain management.

Physical dependence: An adaptive physiological state that can occur with regular drug use and results in withdrawal when drug use is discontinued.

Polydrug abuse: The abuse of two or more drugs at the same time, such as CNS depressant abuse accompanied by abuse of alcohol.

Prescription drug abuse: The intentional misuse of a medication outside of the normally accepted standards of its use.

Prescription drug misuse: Taking a medication in a manner other than that prescribed or for a different condition than that for which the medication is prescribed.

Psychotherapeutics: Drugs that have an effect on the function of the brain and that often are used to treat psychiatric disorders; can include opioids, CNS depressants, and stimulants.

Respiratory depression: Depression of respiration (breathing) that results in the reduced availability of oxygen to vital organs.

Stimulants: Drugs that enhance the activity of the brain and lead to increased heart rate, blood pressure, and respiration; used to treat only a few disorders, such as narcolepsy and attention-deficit hyperactivity disorder.

Tolerance: A condition in which higher doses of a drug are required to produce the same effect as experienced initially.

Tranquilizers: Drugs prescribed to promote sleep or reduce anxiety; this National Household Survey on Drug Abuse classification includes benzodiazepines, barbiturates, and other types of CNS depressants.

Withdrawal: A variety of symptoms that occur after chronic use of some drugs is reduced or stopped.

OTHER HEALTH AND MONEY BOOKS

The following books are offered to our preferred customers at a special price.

BOOK	PRICE
1. Health Secrets	$26.95 *POSTPAID*
2. Money Tips	$26.95 *POSTPAID*
3. The Guidebook of Insiders Tips	$14.95 *POSTPAID*
4. Proven Health Tips Encyclopedia	$17.95 *POSTPAID*
5. Foods That Heal	$19.95 *POSTPAID*
6. Healing & Prevention Secrets	$26.95 *POSTPAID*
7. Most Valuable Book Ever Published	$14.95 *POSTPAID*
8. Book of Home Remedies (hard cover)	$28.95 *POSTPAID*
9. Book of Blood Pressure & Cholestrol	$28.95 *POSTPAID*
10. Good Time Money Book	$26.95 *POSTPAID*
11. Low Price Stocks Newsletter	$99 (12 issues)
12. Penny Stock Profits Newsletterr	$89 (12 issues)

Please send this entire page or write down the names of the books on another sheet of paper and mail it along with your payment .

NAME OF BOOK_____PRICE_____
NAME OF BOOK_____PRICE_____
NAME OF BOOK_____PRICE_____
NAME OF BOOK_____PRICE_____

TOTAL ENCLOSED$_____

SHIP TO:
Name_____
Address_____
City_____ST_____Zip_____

MAIL TO: AMERICAN PUBLISHING CORPORATION
BOOK DISTRIBUTION CENTER
POST OFFICE BOX 15196,
MONTCLAIR, CA 91763-5196